Ready
Set
Heal

A Handbook for Busy Women

A 6-week Plan to Reclaim Your Health and Happiness

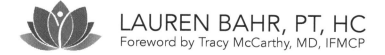

LAUREN BAHR, PT, HC
Foreword by Tracy McCarthy, MD, IFMCP

Ready, Set, Heal: A Handbook for Busy Women
A 6-week plan to reclaim your health and happiness.
By Lauren Bahr, PT, HC

Printed in the United States of America

LCCN: 2018911906

ISBN-13: 978-1727629279
ISBN-10: 1727629272

This book is dedicated to
every woman who desires
better health and happiness.
May this book serve as
your message of hope.

Acknowledgements

Thank you to everyone who helped me with peer reviews and editing. Especially to Beth Hull—your encouragement from day one made this book possible.

Thank you to my husband and kids for your unwavering support. I love you more than you know.

And finally, thank you to my parents for blessing me with a life full of opportunities.

Table of Contents

Foreward

Lauren Bahr and I met for the first time over tea. As a health coach, she was reaching out to me, one of only a few functional medicine doctors in our local community, so she could know a doctor to refer clients to when needed. We connected immediately, sharing the same deep belief in the power of lifestyle and nutrition to transform health.

I may not know you, but I bet I know something about your life, because there is a reason you picked up this book. I know because I have been there, too. Let me see if this describes you: for years you juggled school, friendships, sports, music or other activities, then added a career, relationships. Eventually you added in kids, taking care of the home, keeping in touch with friends, working to keep that spark in your relationship going while your responsibilities at work increased. Now you've taken on leadership positions in your community; maybe you coach soccer now or are the team parent, or you're in the PTA, or you're in charge of the Scouts fundraiser…in other words, you are an expert juggler. You're so good at it, you think nothing of it. You expect it of yourself and think you should be able to handle more. The only problem is, every year there are more balls to keep in the air. Eventually one or more of these balls is going to drop.

At least one of those balls is made of glass, and that is your health.

There are hints that something is wrong: increasing belly fat, fatigue, low energy, nagging digestive issues, brain fog, problems falling asleep or staying asleep, lack of joy even though everything is "fine." Sound familiar? Despite this, you still think of yourself as "healthy." You may even consider these symptoms normal, because so many of your friends have them and they are so common. But common is NOT normal.

It's scary, but these symptoms can be the early signs of chronic disease headed your way. Increasing belly fat can indicate insulin resistance, which can lead to pre-diabetes and diabetes. Sleep problems can mean worsening hormonal imbalances. Digestive issues are a sign of chronic inflammation that can trigger a host of problems, including problems with the health of your brain. And the list goes on.

The number of people with chronic disease is growing at an alarming rate. Currently, 60% of adult Americans have a chronic condition, and 42% have more than one. Autoimmune diseases, digestive disorders, diabetes, Alzheimer's, and other neurodegenerative diseases are all on the rise. Anxiety and depression are also on the rise. Currently, one in six American women are on an antidepressant ("National Center for Health Statistics", 2017). Childhood disease rates are also skyrocketing, including autism, ADHD, anxiety, allergies, and asthma. Our current medical approach to chronic disease has failed. We essentially treat symptoms but not the underlying causes, so the problems progress. These are crippling our health care system, and patients are experiencing a steady decline in quality of life despite medical treatment.

You may be saying, "I've tried to talk to my doctor about my symptoms, but they just say it's normal for my age, or it's normal to experience this after having a baby!" Or maybe your doctor has been sympathetic but didn't have any answers other than a pill. Maybe you tried that pill and it led to side effects.

This isn't your doctor's fault. Our current medical system is a disease management system that is failing people with chronic health conditions. The system was designed for acute care. If you contract a dangerous infection or get seriously injured in a car accident, our medical system is amazing. If you are having a heart attack, you want to be in the hospital. But with chronic disease, we are losing the battle. And that's because we think it is a war!

This battle mindset emerged from fighting serious infectious diseases in the last century, where there was one clear cause for someone's symptoms. But a different mindset is needed to turn the tide of chronic disease. Too often we are locked into looking for a single underlying cause of symptoms because that's the way we've been trained to think, but in doing so, we completely miss the numerous factors adding up to create symptoms.

The answers to relieving the burden of chronic disease lie in looking at traditional cultures and the anthropological record. Research on groups of people living traditional lifestyles, almost identical to their ancestors thousands of years earlier, show us these populations have a startling lack of chronic disease. They show us this profound fact: we are meant to be healthy!

The good news is that we can restore health when we give the body what it needs to heal, the way traditional cultures do. But where do you start? There is endless conflicting dietary information available in books and online. Quick fixes are touted everywhere you look, but anyone who has tried these knows they are disappointing and can lead to other problems. It can be confusing to know where to start. And it may seem downright unbelievable that the simplest changes can produce the most profound effects. But it's true.

The simple but powerful changes outlined in this book work because they realign us with what our bodies expect; they realign us with what we evolved needing: sleep, movement, a clean environment, community, nourishing food, and appropriate levels of stress. We must stop looking for a single cause or cure that we'll never find. Rather, a multitude of factors contribute to the chronic inflammation underlying our symptoms. We must remove the barriers to healing and add in the factors that promote restoration of health.

This approach to treatment is called *functional medicine*. As a physician certified in functional medicine, I look upstream for root causes of your symptoms. In my practice, I use advanced testing to identify system imbalances, such as problems with digestion and absorption, with detoxification or hormones. I identify sources of inflammation and help you remove them. The foundation of treatment in a functional medicine approach is nutritional and lifestyle changes to restore balance to the body's systems and then maintain health. Many people can improve their health dramatically without seeing a functional medicine physician just by making these essential lifestyle changes. Some will get a lot better but need the help of a practitioner to heal the rest of the way. But all the testing in the world won't get you better without laying the foundation, and in this book, Lauren clearly describes the key principles for laying that foundation for healing yourself.

Sound overwhelming? It's actually not. In this wonderful book, Lauren guides you in a step-by-step process to help you make simple changes that will have a deep and lasting impact on your health and your life.

Through applying this approach to my own life and health, I've been able to resolve health challenges and stave off serious issues I was heading towards. In my case, these issues included pre-diabetes, slow but steady weight gain, and a risk of thyroid autoimmune disease that runs in my family. In addition, taking better care of myself now means a smoother transition when menopause comes along and will also keep my brain sharp for decades to come.

You've taken an important step in picking up this book. You are acknowledging there is a problem, and deep down you realize you deserve more—more health, more happiness. The hardest step is to give yourself permission to begin taking care of your health. For us women, this is the real challenge. We serve others constantly. But without self-care, that endless service is unsustainable, and we do a disserve not only to ourselves when we burn out, but to our colleagues and our loved ones.

In this book, Lauren applies her superb health coaching skills in showing you how to begin implementing changes that feel right for you in a way that works with your life. She empathically encourages you to start your healing journey. I've seen Lauren's work with clients firsthand, and her passion and commitment to this approach are inspiring. So, let her inspire and guide you in reclaiming your health so you can live the life you deserve.

Tracy McCarthy, MD, IFMCP
Sacramento, CA
www.catalysthealthcfm.com

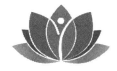

Introduction

If you are reading this book, chances are you are busy, you are tired, and you feel overwhelmed more than you like to admit. Your health has declined, your weight has crept up, and your energy is lacking. You likely have brain fog and maybe you have even lost your "joie de vivre." You want to feel good again, but you are unsure where to start. You are busy and you have an endless to-do list! There's just so much to take care of, right? There are dishes in the sink, the fridge is empty, the floors and bathrooms are dirty again, laundry is piling up, the kids need help with homework, the lawn needs to be mowed, and the list goes on. Your "plate" is full! And there is very little time for YOU.

I can relate all too well. I lived in a constant state of "busy" for many years and it took its toll. In 2014, I felt content and I thought I was thriving. I had a fulfilling career as a physical therapist, a great husband, two beautiful little kids, and a nice home. Life was going along as I had hoped—exactly as I had dreamed of as a little girl. I was living the American Dream. What more could I want?

But things weren't as they seemed. I was tired and burning my candle at both ends. I was depleted. Putting the needs of others before my own, day after day, year after year, made me forget what truly brought me joy. I had lost sight of these things while chasing the American Dream. And then it happened. A perfect storm of additional stress...on top of the stress and depletion that had become my norm.

My level of overwhelm went from mild to severe. I started having trouble sleeping, and without sleep, how could I keep up with my job, my kids, and my endless to-do list? I was scared and I wasn't sure what to do, so I went to the doctor for help. The doctor diagnosed me with depression and anxiety, and she prescribed medication. I was terrified to take the medication because deep down, I didn't believe it was the solution to my problems.

However, I followed the doctor's advice and started medication and talk therapy. But when I went back to my doctor a few weeks later, I was barely holding it together. I was still suffering from insomnia and my stress was through the roof. The doctor looked me in the eyes and suggested I take a medical leave. The thought of taking medical leave was terrifying—I felt like I was being knocked off my pedestal. I felt embarrassed and ashamed of myself for getting to this point. I was worried I would be letting everyone down—my boss, my patients, and my family. But ultimately, I knew the doctor was right. With a heavy heart, I went on medical leave.

Can you imagine being so depleted physically, mentally, and emotionally that you can't work and you barely have the energy to care for your own children? It was terrifying to say the least. I felt like I was letting my kids and my husband down. I was worried about my future and theirs. It seemed like my brain and body were failing me.

At that time, I had very limited understanding of brain health or mental health—and my lack of understanding created a lot of fear. But my education and career as a physical therapist had given me a deep understanding of the body's ability to heal. I had helped thousands of people restore their health. It was my observation that *none* of those people healed from medication alone. I pondered this for my situation and deep down I believed that medication was a temporary band-aid, if it helped at all. I wanted to *truly heal*. The thought of being a depressed and exhausted mom and functioning at anything but my peak potential was not *me*. I had always been a high achiever. I excelled in sports, in school, and I had strong friendships. This new version of me felt foreign.

I am thrilled to report that I have now truly healed. I am the happiest and healthiest I have ever been. In hindsight, I consider this terrifying experience to have been a blessing. My "health crash" was my wake-up call. At the time, I felt broken and scared and I didn't know if I could get better. But what I did know was this: if I limited myself to the western medical approach, I would be medicated for the rest of my life. Think about this…if the medications actually healed the condition they treat, then why do people have to keep taking them their whole lives?

Thankfully, I knew that I had to look outside the proverbial box if I wanted to heal from within. Ultimately, I put myself in the driver's seat and I designed a plan that I hoped would heal my body and mind. I designed this plan based on my observations as a healthcare provider, my basic understanding of nutrition and exercise, and my intuition. My personal prescription included optimizing my nutrition, taking specific supplements, walking daily, doing deep breathing exercises, engaging in guided meditation, prioritizing sleep, participating in talk therapy, and more. In just three months, the dark cloud lifted and I was able to return to work. After one year of devotion to good nutrition and self-care, I felt better than I had in years!

I realized that my tools for healing were actually quite simple, and after transforming my health with these tools, I knew I couldn't keep it a secret. I became determined to share this wisdom to help others. Since 2014, I have voraciously listened to podcasts, read books, learned from top functional medicine experts, and I returned to school to become an Integrative Nutrition Health Coach.

In 2017, in order to fulfill my passion for "being the change I wish to see in the world," I launched my business, Simply Balanced Wellness. As a holistic health coach, I am honored to be helping other women reclaim their health and happiness. I guide my clients to make shifts in their nutrition, lifestyle, and mindset, and the results are amazing. They experience increased energy, weight loss, improved mental clarity, and a renewed sense of joy for life. Additionally, their spouses lose weight and their children have better focus and behavior. These thriving women are creating a ripple effect in their families, workplaces, and communities. I am truly honored to be part of this.

In Part 1 of this book, I will help you get READY to begin your healing journey by teaching you key lessons to unlock your healing potential. In Part 2, you will get SET for your journey by learning the "Nourish to Flourish" toolkit. In Part 3, you will write and implement your own prescription to HEAL. I look forward to hearing how this book improves your health and the health of those around you, too. Let's get started!

"*When sleeping women wake,*

mountains move."

-Chinese Proverb

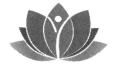

Part 1: Ready

In part 1 of this book you will get ready to heal. You will learn key lessons to unlock your healing potential. These are key lessons that I gathered from a career in conventional healthcare, motherhood, overcoming illness, and discovering functional medicine. Each of these lessons came from epiphanies, or "*aha* moments," in my journey. "*Aha* moments" or "*aha* lessons" are those times when you learn something that you likely already knew, but all of the sudden it clicks and you will never see that situation in the same way again. It is a moment of sudden realization, insight, or deeper understanding. I'm sure you've had moments like this. I've compiled some of my favorite *aha* lessons that I believe will help you shift your view of healing and allow you to change your life in a profoundly positive way.

YOUR BODY IS DESIGNED TO HEAL

Your body is far more capable of healing than you have been led to believe. The human body is designed to heal itself *by itself*. Think back through your life; every cut you have ever had has healed. Every cold and flu you have had, you healed. Your broken bones and muscle strains, those have healed too. Sure, the band-aid provided comfort, the decongestant relieved your stuffy nose, and the cast stabilized your broken bone. These things provided symptom relief, but your body did its own healing in each of these cases.

Somewhere along the way, many of us have forgotten that we have the programming and innate ability to heal. We have been taught that if we are sick, we need to see a doctor. We have been taught that the doctor knows more about our bodies than we do. We have given away our power.

My first job as a physical therapist was at Sinai Hospital in Baltimore, Maryland, where I worked in the Neurorehabilitation Unit. I treated patients who had recently suffered severe strokes or brain injuries. Their deficits were so profound that they were confined to their hospital beds with the exception of their three to four hours of daily rehabilitation (physical therapy, occupational therapy, and speech therapy). This was a dire time for these individuals. Many of them would have died if it weren't for emergency medicine providing life-saving care. The patients who were cognizant were terrified and their loved ones were equally scared and worried.

Thank goodness these patients and their families had access to this wonderful care. This is where our traditional healthcare system shines—with emergency care, trauma care, and acute care. It was during this first job that I witnessed both intense pain and impressive miracles. There were many days I drove home crying because of the heartaches I witnessed in my patients and their families.

I will never forget the twenty-year-old woman who was hit by a car and suffered thirteen fractures, a severe head injury, and multiple lacerated internal organs. Modern medicine saved her life. Surgeons peformed procedures that stopped her internal bleeding and set her bones in a good position for healing. Her complications were so severe that she couldn't speak or get up from the hospital bed for nearly two months. Her first month was spent in the intensive care unit, but at month two, she transferred to inpatient rehabilitation, where I met her.

I worked with her daily for one to two hours. Initially, her physical therapy treatments were very passive; I had to gently move her limbs to provide range of motion to prevent stiffness and bed sores.

Over time, and with the help of two people, she was able to sit at the bedside. And eventually, with my assistance, she was able to stand up from the edge of the bed. By the fourth month, she was able to walk short distances with a walker. Finally, she could be discharged from the hospital and she went home to live with her mother, who was her caregiver and biggest fan. One year later, I visited this young woman and she was smiling and walking normally—she had even started working again! She had made a miraculous recovery and was grateful for her second chance at life. This taught me the power of the body's ability to heal.

I love to observe healing. Most of us in healthcare entered this field because we have a deep passion for helping others. I spent over a decade of my physical therapy career focusing on orthopedics, helping people with joint and muscle pain and dysfunction. I helped countless people recover from back pain, neck pain, rotator cuff tears, carpal tunnel, ACL injuries, ankle sprains, plantar fasciitis, and more. So many of my patients made full recoveries and quickly returned to the activities they loved.

However, not everyone was this fortunate. Over the course of my fifteen years as a physical therapist, I began to notice more and more of my patients had multiple areas of pain. Some of these "pains" had a clear mechanism (e.g. "I twisted my ankle stepping off a curb"), but many did not have a clear injury and they reported that the pain came on gradually. Many of these people were, by definition, suffering from chronic pain. Chronic pain is any pain lasting longer than twelve weeks. Chronic pain is very different from the acute pain you feel when you first sprain your ankle. Acute pain serves a purpose—it's the body's alert system. In the case of an ankle sprain, the pain alerts you to rest and limit movement. Or, if you touch a hot stove, the pain alerts you to remove your hand as quickly as possible to prevent a worse burn. Acute pain is normal. Chronic pain, while common, is *not* normal.

As a healthcare provider, I could not ignore the increasing percentage of patients I was seeing with chronic pain. It is one thing for an eighty-year-old woman with a lifetime of wear and tear and forward head posture to have chronic neck pain and stiff shoulders. But I was noticing people in their seventies, sixties, fifties, forties, thirties and even in their twenties with chronic pain! This shocked me and it was heartbreaking to see. These patients of mine struggled each day to do their daily activities, and many had lost the ability to do what they once loved to do. Some had severe pain, but even those with low grade persistent pain were left feeling drained and irritable. This made me wonder why these people were suffering. Why hadn't their bodies healed? I was seeing the same pattern with regard to chronic disease—more and more patients of all ages were being diagnosed with chronic conditions—autoimmune diseases, neurodegenerative diseases, depression, and more.

Why are we having an epidemic of chronic pain and chronic disease? Millions of people suffering with chronic pain and chronic disease are turning to their doctors for help. Western medicine is diagnosing their conditions and then medicating these people to suppress their symptoms. But it is missing the *why*. Why are these people hurting? Why are they suffering with chronic health conditions? Why are they not healing? This question was slapping me in the face each day I went to work as a physical therapist. I could no longer ignore it.

INFLAMMATION IS AT THE ROOT OF MOST ILLNESSES:

I wanted answers as to why people were suffering with chronic pain and chronic illness. In my quest for deeper understanding, I started listening to podcasts, watching TED talks, and reading books that challenged the currently accepted belief systems of health and wellness that I'd been indoctrinated with during my conventional training.

A real eye-opener for me was reading the book *Grain Brain* by Dr. David Perlmutter. I learned that our Standard American Diet was a huge factor contributing to chronic diseases related to the brain and the body. Shortly thereafter I watched the TED talk by Dr. Terry Wahls where she explains how she put her multiple sclerosis (MS) into remission after many years of decline and being confined to a motorized wheelchair. She restored her ability to walk and even ride a bike—mostly through dietary changes! This was unheard of in my career thus far. Any patient I had seen with MS was declining as time ticked by. After all, it is a "progressive neurogenerative disease."

Within that book and TED talk, I had finally found an answer to why some of my patients were getting stuck in a state of chronic pain and chronic disease. The Standard American Diet (AKA the "SAD diet") and our modern lifestyle are highly inflammatory. It turns out that inflammation is at the root of most chronic disease and chronic pain.

This concept of systemic (or full-body) inflammation was new to me. In my physical therapy education I had learned about inflammation and how it is the body's normal response after an injury. How could a "normal" physiological response go awry? Stay with me for a quick explanation…

Your body has an innate ability to heal itself. You have an immune system that helps you fight infection, bacteria and disease. Your immune system also helps you heal from injuries. Think back to a time when you sprained your ankle or slammed your finger in a door—during these *acute* injuries, your body responded with pain, heat, swelling, redness, and temporary loss of function of that body part. These are the hallmark signs of inflammation. This *normal* response to injury is necessary for proper healing in a healthy individual. Broken bones heal within six to eight weeks, and mild soft tissue injuries (like ankle sprains and pulled muscles) heal within a few weeks. Severe soft tissue injuries (like those associated with trauma) generally heal within twelve weeks. But some people have pain that lasts beyond this twelve-week mark, and we label them with "chronic pain." My question was *why* did chronic pain happen to this sub-group of individuals?

Here was my *aha* moment: These individuals are often in a state of chronic inflammation. Chronic inflammation creates persistent irritation and swelling inside the body, in any region, even in the brain! Many of the patients I was seeing who were stuck with chronic pain had chronic inflammation as an underlying factor. (Please note, chronic pain is complex and I'm not claiming that inflammation is the only factor; however, it is an important factor to consider.)

I went on to learn that medical researchers and functional medicine doctors agree that chronic inflammation plays a role not only in chronic pain, but also in *most* of the chronic diseases we face as a nation. Chronic inflammation plays a role in asthma, heart disease, diabetes, obesity, certain cancers, adrenal fatigue, rheumatoid arthritis, lupus, multiple sclerosis, Hashimotos, Parkinson's disease, IBS, depression, anxiety, Alzheimer's, autism, and more! If you or a loved one has a diagnosis on this list, then this book is full of actionable steps that you can take to reduce *chronic systemic inflammation*. Reducing inflammation through better nutrition and lifestyle choices may be the missing link to improving your health and happiness.

Why hasn't your doctor told you this? It's quite possible your doctor doesn't know this information and even if he or she knows, it doesn't change the approach to care that they were taught. Conventional medicine is focused on symptom suppression. If you have pain, your doctor prescribes a pain medication. If you have acid reflux, your doctor prescribes an acid blocker. If you have an autoimmune disease, your doctor prescribes an immunosuppressive medication. While ibuprofen and other NSAIDs (nonsteroidal anti-inflammatories), as well as steroid medications, have powerful anti-inflammatory effects, and while they have their place in trauma and acute injury care, they are not designed for long-term use. Please note that *no* drug is without side effects. Often people on prescription medications end up taking additional medications to combat the side effects of the first medication they are taking. This is known as poly-pharmacy. The primary tool in the western medicine "toolbox" is pharmaceutical drugs. Your conventional doctor is trained to match a drug to your symptoms. But the problem with this approach is that it usually fails to address the underlying causes of the symptoms.

I'm excited to tell you that there is a different approach—one that has few side effects and the potential for amazing benefits. Even if you don't have one of the previously mentioned diagnoses, you may have nagging symptoms related to chronic inflammation. According to Dr. Susan Blum's *The Immune System Recovery Plan,* "Inflammation can cause a wide range of symptoms, including fatigue, puffiness, muscle or joint pain, abdominal discomfort including diarrhea, and difficulty concentrating or 'brain fog.' Or you may just have a vague, nagging feeling that something isn't right, even if your doctor can't find anything wrong with you" (Blum, 2013, p. 14). Do you have any of those symptoms?

Now that you know inflammation is an underlying factor in your current health conditions, the next question is *why* are you experiencing inflammation? There are *many* ontributing factors.

Factors that increase inflammation:

- The highly inflammatory Standard American Diet (SAD diet)—sugar, gluten, dairy, and processed foods

- Physical stress—injuries, infections, surgeries, intense physical labor, or overexertion

- Emotional stress—related to relationships, jobs, and negative thought patterns

- Toxins--environmental toxins, chemicals in household and beauty products, pesticides in and on food, and heavy metal exposure

Part II and Part III of this book will empower you to make changes in these areas that will reduce your levels of chronic systemic inflammation.

SHIFT AWAY FROM TREATING DISEASE TO INSTEAD CREATING HEALTH

Imagine you walk into your kitchen and you see that your sink is overflowing. What do you do? Do you grab a towel and throw it on the floor? And if one towel is not enough, do you grab every towel in the house to mop up the overflow? *Or*, do you instead ask, "Why is the sink overflowing?"

I think you would ask why! You would then figure it out—the sink is overflowing because it's full of dishes and someone (your pesky toddler?) left the water running. Your solution is to turn off the water. And voila, the water stops overflowing. You have corrected the problem at its source.

Let's apply this analogy to medical care. If you have a headache, you were likely taught to take ibuprofen or aspirin. If you experience chronic and severe headaches, your doctor may have prescribed a stronger medication. You are now taking this medication several times each week. (This is like throwing more towels on the floor without addressing the cause of the overflow). But why are you getting these headaches in the first place? Sure, maybe you had bloodwork done, but did you or the doctor seek out the underlying cause of your headaches? I realize this is a complex topic, but I know many women firsthand who have reversed their severe headaches (even migraines) through nutrition and lifestyle changes. For some of them, gluten was the underlying cause; for others it was a combination of stressors in their life (lack of sleep along with work stress and dehydration, and so on). When these women re-moved gluten and/or improved their self-care and lifestyle factors, their headaches resolved. Once they corrected the problem upstream, they no longer needed to suppress symptoms downstream.

So, instead of throwing towels on the floor when your sink is overflowing, seek to understand *why* the overflow is happening in the first place and correct the problem at the source.

By now, I've explained that the traditional medical model often treats disease by suppressing symptoms. You go to the doctor and you tell them your chief complaints (your symptoms). The doctor then performs an exam (collects signs). The doctor assesses your signs and symptoms and gives you a diagnosis (a label). The doctor then prescribes a drug based on your diagnosis. The meds are designed to suppress your symptoms. But in this model, the *why* behind the symptoms is often missed. Drugs are merely one approach to managing disease. Sometimes drugs are necessary, but often there are other great options once you become open to them.

In functional medicine and in holistic health coaching, we shift away from treating the disease or label. Instead, we focus on building health for the individual. It's possible that you have been led to believe that once something in your body is "broken," you then have to live that way forever. This is often not true. Again, your body is designed to heal. When we focus on creating health through improved nutrition and lifestyle, surprising changes begin to happen.

Here's a story to illustrate my point. A thirty-three-year-old woman, Kate (name changed to protect her privacy) came to see me. She was suffering from severe chronic back pain, describing it as a ten out of ten on the pain chart. Also, her hands and feet were swollen and stiff, and covered with eczema. She was scared about the pain, embarrassed about the rashes, and sad that her health conditions made it difficult to care for her toddler.

Because of my medical background, I had a strong suspicion that she had an undiagnosed autoimmune condition. She did report that she had recently seen a rheumatologist and had some diagnostic testing done—she was meeting with that doctor in two weeks to find out her results and diagnosis. But she was ready to make changes in the meantime—especially if there was something that could help her. I suggested a specific nutrition plan to help reduce her inflammation.

She implemented the dietary changes right away. Within two weeks, her pain was lowered to five out of ten. After four weeks of following the nutrition and lifestyle recommendations I gave her, the pain was reduced to two out of ten, and her eczema had resolved completely! She felt great and was able to care for her child again.

As suspected, the rheumatologist diagnosed her with psoriatic arthritis. At the time of writing this, Kate has never taken the prescribed immune-suppressing drugs—she hasn't needed to! It has been one year since she first came to me. During this time she has shed over twenty-five pounds, she continues to follow an anti-inflammatory diet, she is free from pain and eczema, and she is active and playful with her toddler. Her rheumatologist is amazed that her bloodwork indicates extremely low levels of inflammation—this doctor has never seen a case like this before.

Kate reversed many of her symptoms within one month. And as we continued to work together, she also began seeing a functional medicine doctor—with this combination of care, Kate has successfully put her autoimmune disease into remission!

Instead of suppressing your nagging health symptoms, I want you to shift to a framework of creating health. The more you nourish your body, the more it will do what it is brilliantly designed to do--heal itself *by itself*. The keys to unlock that healing are changes to your nutrition, lifestyle, and mindset—all of which I will teach you in Part 2 of this book. But for now, I have a few more *aha* lessons to share with you.

YOUR GENES ARE NOT YOUR DESTINY

*"Your genetics load the gun.
Your lifestyle pulls the trigger."*

-Dr. Mehmet Oz

Your genes predispose you to certain conditions, but there's no guarantee that you will develop them. For example, if your mom has rheumatoid arthritis and your dad died from cancer, then you may have genetic factors that predispose you to these diseases, but it does not mean that you will develop them.

In 2018, Dr. Ben Lynch published a groundbreaking book titled *Dirty Genes*. In this book he discusses the power of epigenetics and he shares ways to optimize your health by optimizing your genetic expression. What is epigenetics? This is an emerging area of research looking at the ability for genes to be turned on or off, or "expressed." There are many factors that can influence this expression. Dr. Lynch writes that, "…we can transform our genetic destiny through a combination of diet, supplements, sleep, stress relief, and reduced exposure to environmental toxins (the toxins in our food, water, air, and products)." (Lynch, 2018, p. 2)

Perhaps you already have an autoimmune disease, or diabetes, or a diagnosed digestive condition. You may believe that you will have the related symptoms for the rest of your life, and that the best you can do is manage the symptoms with medications and accept your condition. Well, this may or *may not* be the case, depending on your situation. Like me and my clients, you might be able to reverse your symptoms—even those you have lived with for many years. This is why I love sharing the power of nutrition and lifestyle changes. The story I shared earlier about Kate is a perfect example of reversing a chronic health condition—an autoimmune condition that most people will suffer ill-effects from for the rest of their lives—both from the disease and from the medication side effects. Kate was able to influence her genetic expression in a positive way through a combination of health coaching and functional medicine.

In the introduction, I shared the story of my health crash in 2014. When I sought medical care, I was led to believe that I would have these conditions for the rest of my life and the best I could do was manage the symptoms with medication. Fortunately, I listened to my intuition and decided to use nutrition and lifestyle to my advantage. I was fortunate to have already discovered the concept of chronic systemic inflammation. It made sense that it was an underlying cause of chronic disease and chronic pain.

At that time, I had limited knowledge of depression and anxiety, but thankfully I had listened to a podcast interview at one point along the way that mentioned the concept of brain inflammation--that it was a major factor in depression and anxiety. The term "brain-flammation" had stuck in my head from that podcast episode. I felt a glimmer of hope that if I could reduce my systemic and brain inflammation, then maybe I could recover.

I wasn't sure what gains I could make, but I knew I had nothing to lose by taking better care of my body. And that's when I wrote my own personal prescription. I made a checklist and followed it diligently each day. It included: walking for ten minutes, barefoot yoga for five minutes, deep breathing, guided meditation, eating nutrient-dense foods, taking a few specific supplements, prioritizing my sleep, and tapping into my support network of family, friends, and trusted therapist. What I didn't know at that time was that my health crash was actually my wake-up call—my opportunity to make radical changes in my life and experience profound and deep healing. As I mentioned earlier, it took three months for me to heal to the point where I could return to work. After one year of devotion to self-care, I felt better than I had in years.

After healing myself through holistic means, I went on to help my husband and my child reverse their chronic health conditions. For the first ten years I'd known my husband, he suffered from allergies. He was allergic to pets, dust, pollen, and more. Over time, he also developed asthma. His evenings and weekends were often spent with a box of tissues in hand, and by Sunday, it was like his immune system had had enough and he would spend the day on the sofa, sneezing and blowing his nose. He blamed it on the cat and dog and recounted that his allergies had started as a young child. It was something he had just learned to live with. Daily allergy meds and daily inhalers were his norm. He believed he would have allergies and asthma for the rest of his life.

Fortunately, he made nutritional changes with me. When I decided to go gluten-free, he agreed that the entire family could do a one-month trial together. When I started buying more organic foods, he supported it completely. As a family, we began eating more nutrient-dense foods and less processed junk. Within one month of going gluten-free, my husband noticed a drastic reduction in his allergy symptoms. It was significant enough that he has chosen to remain gluten free ever since. With my assistance and guidance from an excellent naturopathic doctor, my husband followed a gut healing program. The results are amazing--he no longer suffers from the frequent allergy attacks, asthma, and headaches that plagued him for years! Instead, he enjoys good health, better energy, more productive workdays, and fun-filled evenings and weekends with our family. Additionally, he has been able to discontinue his use of all medications and inhalers.

My children have also benefitted from our improved nutrition and lifestyle choices. My son had suffered from eczema since he was a baby. As a toddler, he was often constipated and said, "My body hurts," which was his way of saying that his stomach ached. Once we removed gluten from our diets, it took only *three days* for his eczema to resolve completely. The stomach aches and some of his other health issues took a bit longer to figure out. We eventually worked with a naturopathic doctor and then a functional medicine doctor. Through nutrition and lifestyle changes combined with specific supplementation (guided by functional medicine test results), he has experienced radical improvements in his health.

Through my personal experience—for myself, my family and my clients—I have witnessed health recoveries that some may call "miracles." Maybe they are, but maybe each of us has influenced our epigenetics in a positive way through nutrition and lifestyle factors. I have heard numerous similar health recovery testimonials from my health coach and functional medicine colleagues.

Recovery is possible for many people suffering from depression, anxiety, chronic pain, autoimmunity, diabetes, cancer, and more. Your genes do not have to be your destiny.

ALL DISEASE BEGINS IN THE GUT

"All disease begins in the gut."

-Hippocrates

Hippocrates lived from 460 BC to 370 BC and he is often referred to as "the father of modern medicine." He is also famous for saying, "Let food be thy medicine and thy medicine be thy food." Interestingly, his theories were forgotten for many years, but they are re-surfacing in a big way. Gut health and good nutrition are becoming popular again--as they should be.

I can say with certainty that gut health and nutrition never came up in my formal physical therapy education or in my fifteen-year career in healthcare (and I took at least thirty hours of continuing education every two years). It was when I learned about Dr. Terry Wahls and her amazing recovery from multiple sclerosis, where she used food as medicine, that I began to understand what Hippocrates was talking about. Since her recovery, Dr. Wahls has become a leader in the area of functional medicine. Functional medicine is built on the foundation that disease begins in the gut and therefore healing also begins in the gut.

What exactly is the gut? The gut refers to the human digestive tract. A healthy digestive system extracts calories and nutrients from your food. It also detoxifies and eliminates waste. But there is a lot more to the story, because the gut is home to a complex ecosystem that contains trillions of bacterial cells, both good and bad ones. These bacteria, plus fungi and viruses, live in your digestive tract and are known as the microbiome. The microbiome has direct communication with your brain via a nerve called the vagus nerve. I was surprised to learn that most of our serotonin (the feel-good neurotransmitter) is made in the gut. And, also of utmost importance, at least seventy percent of your immune system is located in the walls of the gut! Yes, a healthy gut is essential for health and happiness.

Unfortunately, with our modern diet and lifestyle choices, the microbiome and the gut become damaged. Many people have inadequate good bacteria and excessive harmful bacteria. This leads to an imbalance of gut flora (an imbalance known as dysbiosis) and increased permeability of the intestinal walls (known as "leaky gut"). In a leaky gut, the intestinal membrane "holes" become larger and allow food particles (versus just nutrients) and bacteria to leak into the bloodstream, which creates chronic systemic inflammation. Research supports that inflammation from leaky gut is linked to hundreds of symptoms and diseases. The symptoms may be related to digestion, such as constipation, gas, diarrhea, or bloating. Or, they may show up as joint stiffness, pain, seasonal allergies, asthma, mood disorders, brain fog, food allergies, and/or rashes.

Basically, poor gut health results in poor general health.

There are many factors that negatively influence gut health. The SAD (Standard American Diet) is a big factor because it lacks essential nutrients *and* is full of inflammatory sugar, pesticides that damage the gut walls, and antibiotics from factory-farmed animal protein that kill the good gut bacteria. Stress has become pervasive in our culture and this is another factor that damages gut health.

Factors that contribute to gut dysbiosis and leaky gut:

- The SAD diet
- Overuse of medications (including antibiotics, NSAIDs, birth control, antacids, etc.)
- Chronic stress
- Environmental toxins (in the air, beauty products, household chemicals, and more)

If this is new information for you, it can feel difficult and overwhelming to learn about. Please keep in mind that knowledge is power. You have the ability to make different choices moving forward. The steps outlined in this book will provide many strategies for improving your gut health. Better gut health creates a stronger immune system and better production of serotonin and other feel-good neurotransmitters. Each step in the right direction is worth it.

LEAD YOUR JOURNEY

*"When writing the story of your life,
don't let anyone else hold the pen."*

-Unknown

Do you let others hold the pen in your life story? I meet many women who are living their lives on autopilot. Day after day, they perform the tasks they believe they *should* do and often neglect what they *want* to do. Do you feel a sense of control in your life? Some people feel like someone else, or their job, controls their life. If you are lacking a sense of control, it can create a huge amount of stress. This stress has a negative effect on your health and happiness (and microbiome, as we discussed earlier).

In observing thousands of patients during my career as a physical therapist, I became fascinated with why some people healed and why others didn't. There are of course many factors, but one thing that became evident is that people who lacked a sense of control often had poor outcomes. These people often felt like victims of their circumstance and they were relying on an external person or pill to "fix" them. This is known as an external locus of control.

Conversely, my patients who felt in control of their choices and took ownership and responsibility for healing often had better outcomes. This is known as an internal locus of control. These individuals sought advice from the doctor and me (as their physical therapist), then they took medications they believed would help them, *and* they took responsibility for their self-care.

As a physical therapist I helped rehabilitate hundreds of people after total knee replacement surgery. Those who had an internal locus of control followed their self-care program and generally excelled. They took responsibility and did their exercises as prescribed and applied ice with elevation as prescribed. They restored their knee motion within a month and they returned to their normal daily activities within a few months, on schedule. Conversely, those patients who were "non-compliant" with their exercises and ice routine became stiff and had a prolonged recovery and/or poor outcomes—meaning some of them struggled to restore normal walking and daily activities. Of course, there are often many confounding variables for each person and each situation, but I observed this trend more often than not. The people with an internal locus of control took responsibility for their self-care and believed that it made a difference in their outcome, and it usually did.

When my health crashed in 2014, I used this information to my advantage. I knew that I had to adopt an internal locus of control. I could not wait for some outside force to fix me. There was no doctor or pill that could fix the stressors in my life and the anxiety and fatigue I was experiencing. Instead, I wrote my personal prescription and followed it daily. If I cheated, I was only cheating myself. I literally made myself a checklist and each day I diligently accomplished each task. Some items on the list took one minute, others took ten or twenty minutes. But I did them each day, because if I didn't, then who would? I believe that taking ownership in my healing journey was essential to my recovery.

In working with my health coaching clients, I help them foster an internal locus of control. I can be their coach and teach, encourage, support, and hold them accountable, but ultimately, they are the ones making positive habit changes in the areas of nutrition and self-care. One obstacle that I encounter is that many of these women feel that they lack discipline, and therefore, they have a difficult time making positive habit changes. Do you sometimes feel this too? Take a moment to think about this—have you ever promised yourself that you would do something (such as exercise) and then fail to do so? If yes, you are not alone, because we have all been there. But if this is chronically your situation, then what is at the root of your lack of self-discipline? Is it lack of belief that your effort will pay off? Or could it be lack of self-love? (I bring this up because it is more common than you realize). Why do you feel you aren't worth taking time to care for yourself? Yes, it's important to take care of your kids. Yes, it's important to take care of your home. Yes, it's important to give your work your best effort. But at the end of the day, who's taking care of *you*?

Think about when you're on an airplane—the flight

attendant gives that instructional talk before the plane takes off and tells you that if the cabin loses oxygen pressure, masks will drop from the ceiling. If you're flying with a young child, who do you put the oxygen mask on first? I hope you put it on yourself. If you put it on your child first, you could pass out in the meantime! The same is true in life—if you're running around putting oxygen masks on everybody else, how do you expect to survive, or even thrive? If you're like me, sometimes it's helpful to be reminded of how essential self-care is. In Part II and Part III of this book, you'll identify simple actionable steps for putting oxygen on you first. You have my full permission to love and take care of you.

Self-care allows you to share the best of you, rather than what is left of you.

I encourage you to keep an open mind as you read this book. Try to figure out what action steps you can take to restore your health. Take hold of the pen that tells your life story; take full responsibility and make your health and happiness a priority. You will benefit, and so will everyone around you. You are worth it.

And if you're a person who needs accountability, I will teach you how to build that into your personal prescription. Most of us need accountability, and that's okay. Perhaps you have tried to have discipline but you're not getting the results you expected. Maybe you've tried to cut out sugar, only to end up back on the sugar addiction bandwagon. Or maybe you're cutting calories and exercising in an attempt to lose weight, but you're left feeling hungry and irritable and still unable to lose weight.

These situations are common and frustrating. Many of my health coaching clients have experienced this before they start my program. I was there once, too. Sugar is highly addictive, and weight loss is often difficult. We have been confused by all the contradictory diets and misinformation out there.

Part 2 of this book will give you clarity so that you can overcome these challenges once and for all. Many of the concepts will be a review of what you already know, but others will require you to replace some of your current beliefs about nutrition and self-care.

CREATE A HEALING TEAM

*"We don't have to do all of it alone.
We were never meant to."*

-Brené Brown (writer, speaker, research professor)

Yes, you are responsible for leading your healing journey, but keep in mind you don't have to do it alone. In fact, I encourage you to find support. I like to call such a support network a "healing team."

Healing teams are very important. I recently had a consultation with a potential client who wanted to begin my health coaching program. In talking to her, I could see that she was highly motivated and a good match for my program. However, I could also see that she had some deep emotional pain that was surfacing as we spoke. I agreed to work with her, but I also suggested that she work with a trained psychotherapist concurrently. I gave her some options for seeking therapy and she promptly scheduled a visit with a therapist for the following week. I was impressed with her initiative and her ability to act.

My goal in suggesting a therapist for her was to create a healing team. She also expressed that she had good support from her husband and her mother in seeking an integrative approach for her recovery. Your team may include a health coach, a functional medicine doctor, a physical therapist, a psychotherapist, a massage therapist, or any other healer(s) of your choice. There is so much to learn from different healers, but ultimately you get to be the decision maker in your journey.

It's also helpful to have your spouse and at least one friend who support the changes you're making to better your health. Therefore, your healing team can be any combination of professionals, friends, and family.

You are responsible for your choices and new habits, but having a supportive healing team can make a huge difference in your success.

FIXER VS. FACILITATOR

As a young physical therapist in my twenties, trained in the traditional western medical model of care, I believed that I was healing my patients. When patients came to me with back pain, I evaluated them and provided appropriate care including therapeutic massage, education about their condition, heat with electrical stimulation, etc. After a handful of visits, most of them were feeling better. It was very rewarding—they were happy, and I was happy. But some people with back pain didn't get better and I found that I would blame myself. I questioned whether I had performed the techniques correctly. I questioned whether I needed to take more continuing education. I began to doubt my abilities because I believed that I was supposed to "fix" them.

Over time, I learned that my patients and I were a team. I made this clear to them. "We are a team. Here's what I can do to help you. Here's what I need you to do to facilitate the process between visits." I was no longer a "fixer;" instead I became a "facilitator." This was a much more effective model of care!

Your healthcare providers are not fixers; they are facilitators.

Your doctor (or other health care provider) is *not* fixing you. They're facilitating your healing journey. It is your body that is healing itself. Always. This is an important key point--one that you need to know in order to reclaim your health and happiness. A good facilitator will feel like a good fit and will accelerate your journey.

At the beginning of my healing journey, my facilitators and healing team included: a doctor, a therapist, my husband, and a few close friends. I was in charge of the choices I made, but each of them provided a unique pillar of support.

More recently, I have chosen to work with a mindset coach and a tapping therapist—my goal is to be the best version of me so that I can bring that forward to be a better mom, wife, family member, friend, and health coach. Working on *me* has allowed me to get to this point in my life so that I can share this book with you.

KEY POINTS FROM PART 1:

1. Your body is designed to heal, and it is far more capable of healing than you have been led to believe.

2. Inflammation is often at the root of chronic health conditions.

3. Shift away from treating disease. Instead, focus on creating health.

4. Your genes are not your destiny. Your nutrition and lifestyle choices impact your genetic expression.

5. All disease begins in the gut and therefore all healing begins in the gut.

6. Be in control of your journey. Take full responsibility for your choices moving forward.

7. Create a healing team.

8. Remember that your healthcare providers are "facilitators" and not "fixers."

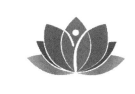

Part 2: Set

In Part 2, you'll learn of six key areas to nourish your body and mind so that you can ignite your innate healing potential. The steps to take in these areas comprise what I like to call the "nourish to flourish toolkit." There is also a special section for moms and a special section for women with anxiety.

As you know, millions of women struggle with low energy, brain fog, anxiety, depression, digestive issues, and difficulty losing weight. Unfortunately, these symptoms are *very* common. According to the National Institute of Health, more than two out of three adults are overweight ("Over-weight & Obesity Statistics", 2017). According to the CDC (Centers for Disease Control and Prevention), one out of six adult women in the US is taking prescription antidepressants ("National Center for Health Statistics", 2017). But "common" does *not* mean "normal." As I have previously explained, your body is designed to heal and to be healthy.

In the past, I viewed symptoms as something that I needed to "make go away." But over time, I have shifted my viewpoint. Instead, I now view symptoms as signals from the body. Just as your car has a check engine light and a gas light, your body has built-in feedback systems. If your gas light turns on, you know you need to get gas. If you ignore it or put black tape over the light, it doesn't change the fact that you need gas. This is similar for your body. If you are tired, it doesn't mean that you need more coffee or more sugary foods to stimulate energy. Instead, feeling fatigued is like a warning light. If you dial in the quality of your nutrition, sleep, joy, and thought patterns, there's a good chance you will experience an increase in energy. And this isn't rocket science. I'm here to remind you that you already know far more about optimizing your health than you realize.

One problem is that in today's fast-paced world, we have become accustomed to wanting "faster, better, more"—also known as instant gratification. There is not one single "right" way to heal, but there are wrong ways. One wrong way is to pop a pill with the expectation that it will fix you. As I mentioned earlier, there is a time and place for medication, but for chronic health conditions, medication will not fix you. It may suppress a symptom, but it fails to address the root cause of the dysfunction. For a deeper dive to learn when drugs are necessary and when alternatives are better, please read the book *Mind Over Meds* by Dr. Andrew Weil.

Read on to discover my Nourish to Flourish Toolkit, a framework for healing your body and mind that are based on functional medicine principles. As you provide nourishment in these six areas, you will begin to see a positive shift in your health and happiness.

I encourage you to keep an open mind as you read through this section of the book. Some of the information will seem contradictory to what you have been conditioned to think, believe, and do. If you really pause and think about this information, I suspect you will find that it intuitively makes sense. Again, keep an open mind and *get set* to begin your healing journey.

NOURISH TO FLOURISH TOOLKIT:

- Nourish with Food
- Nourish with Water
- Nourish with Sleep
- Nourish with Movement
- Nourish with Mindset
- Nourish with Joy

NOURISH WITH FOOD

"Nothing tastes as good as being healthy feels."

-Unknown

Entire books are devoted to the topic of nutrition. In fact, there are hundreds of different books covering nutrition, and yet they are all different and sometimes share contradictory information! So, if you are feeling confused about what to eat or which diet to follow, you are not alone.

I was confused for *many* years. It wasn't until I attended the Institute for Integrative Nutrition (IIN) when I had to learn one hundred dietary theories that things finally clicked. Prior to IIN, I was already on a quest to eat well. I had completed an elimination diet (a short-term eating plan to eliminate certain foods that might be causing allergies or other symptoms), and I had already begun to discover a style of eating that worked well for me.

By doing a four-week elimination diet, I had learned that gluten and dairy were triggers for some of my health issues including brain fog, constipation, and acne. I had learned that a gluten- and dairy-free diet rich in protein, healthy fats, veggies, and gluten-free grains was ideal for me--but was it the perfect diet for everyone? Here's the answer: NO. There is not one single perfect human diet. I am not going to tell you to switch to one hundred percent paleo or one hundred percent vegetarian, because I don't know your unique health history and I don't know which dietary plan is best suited for your unique dietary needs.

When I work one-on-one with my clients, I can give more specific and customized advice; however, for the purpose of this book, I will teach you a way of eating that will boost your nutrient intake, reduce your intake of toxins, and reduce your inflammation. There are some common denominators that work well for most people, but the term *"bio-individuality"** applies here. Bio-individuality means that we each have unique nutritional needs; we each must listen our bodies and intuition to discover which foods work best for us.

The term "bio-individuality"

The Institute for Integrative Nutrition® teaches the term "bio-individuality", which is the concept that no one diet or lifestyle works for everyone. Each person's nutritional needs are individual, and based on a number of varying factors such as lifestyle, occupation, climate, age, gender, culture, and religion. Lifestyle needs are individual as well; what works for one person may not work for another with regard to relationships, exercise, career, spirituality, and physical activity. Additionally, people's needs change over time, so it is important to check in with yourself as you evolve.

© Integrative Nutrition Inc. | Integrative Nutrition Inc. does not endorse the content contained in this book

Earlier in the book, we discussed that inflammation is the root cause of most chronic health conditions. I also mentioned that there are multiple causes of inflammation, including the SAD diet, stress, and toxins. I believe that changing your diet is one of the most powerful ways to reduce your inflammation.

The highly inflammatory SAD diet includes excessive amounts of processed foods, junk oils, gluten, dairy, and sugar. These foods tend to increase inflammation in your body and lead to weight gain. Even if you are very physically active, you cannot out-exercise the SAD diet.

"You can't exercise your way out of a bad diet."

-Mark Hyman, MD

Additionally, it can be difficult to have proper energy for exercise if you are eating the SAD diet. Food is fuel for the body. When you provide the body with the correct fuel, it runs efficiently. Your fuel, or food, comes in the form of three main macro-nutrients: fats, protein, and carbohydrates. Each person will need differing amounts of these macronutrients, but all three are necessary.

Clearly, there have been many dietary fads that have

come and gone. During the 1990s, our nation was led to believe that eating fat made people fat. As a result, most of us switched to a low-fat or fat-free diet and guess what happened? Obesity, diabetes, and chronic disease skyrocketed! Did you gain weight during the low-fat era? I sure did! I became a "pro" at eating low-fat foods. I ate my bagel with low-fat cream cheese for breakfast, a sandwich with fat-free deli meat and fat-free cheese for lunch, and fat-free pasta with marinara sauce for dinner. I snacked on fat-free cookies and "gummy candies," and guess what happened? I got fat! I was thirty pounds heavier than I am now. Not only that, I was constantly tired and craving sweets; it was like I had no "off switch" when it came to eating, and I was uncomfortable in my own body. My diet at that time consisted predominately of two things: carbohydrates and sugar. Carbohydrates in the body are broken down into sugar. Sugar plus more sugar is a recipe for inflammation which leads to weight gain, diabetes, skin problems, hormonal issue, mood issues and more!

Excess carbohydrates and sugar are making you fat (and sick).

In his book *Eat Fat, Get Thin,* Dr. Mark Hyman, a functional medicine doctor and public figure, discusses the science behind why your body and brain need fat. I highly recommend his book. He has very well-researched and sound nutrition advice. What I will continue to share in this section jives with his recommendations—as well as the recommendations of many other functional medicine experts out there.

Not all calories are created equal.

In my college Nutrition 101 class, I learned about the macronutrients I previously mentioned--fats, protein, and carbohydrates. I also learned about calories. The message I took away from that class was that if I reduced my caloric intake and exercised more, then I would lose weight. Do you believe this too? Most Americans (even most doctors) believe that this is true. If this were true, and it were this simple, then weight loss would be easy for people!

But you and I both know that weight loss is challenging--more difficult than that simple formula. Hormones, neurotransmitters, gut health, and emotions all come into play. Also, eating 2,000 calories of junk food during the course of your day feels very different from eating 2,000 calories of veggies, lean protein, healthy fats, whole grains, and fresh fruit. This is because food carries information to each cell of your body; that information is in the form of nutrients, vitamins, and minerals. The types of foods you eat impact your hormones, gut health, immune system, metabolism, and weight.

In the world of health coaching and functional medicine, we say that "food is information" because the food you eat becomes assimilated by your body during the process of digestion. Your food becomes your blood, which becomes your cells, which make up your organs, which make up you! I'm pretty sure you want to be "made" of high quality, nutrient-dense, whole foods. You do not want to be composed of nutrient-depleted fast food or high-sugar junk foods.

To properly nourish with food, you will want to eliminate foods that are inflammatory and you will want to consume foods that carry essential vitamins and minerals for your body (and brain) to heal and thrive. Which foods increase inflammation? This can vary, depending on the person and their unique situation, but here are the top offenders.

Top inflammatory foods:
- Sugar
- Processed foods (aka "chemicalized junk food")
- Gluten
- Dairy (for some people)
- Junk oils

Sugar and processed foods are highly addictive and they create inflammation in the body. Removing sugar and processed foods (or reducing them to a very small portion of your diet) will likely have a huge impact on your health. Sugar is toxic to the body and is a key contributor to obesity, diabetes, heart disease, and some cancers. Processed foods typically contain sugar, as well as chemicals and artificial substances which are not really even food! I am not a hundred percent sugar free—I enjoy indulging in dark chocolate and occasional "sweet treats," but sugar makes up a very small percentage of what I eat.

Gluten is also inflammatory and negatively affects

your gut health. Gluten is a protein found in wheat, barley, and rye. Gluten-filled products in your home include: cereal, bread, pasta, crackers, cookies, cakes, waffles, and more. I suggest that you get into the habit of reading labels to make sure the food does not contain wheat, barley, or rye. Also, it's best for the label to have a short ingredient list that includes items that you know are food.

There are entire books devoted to the topic of gluten—one I suggest you read is *Grain Brain* by David Perlmutter, MD. Why is gluten a problem? There are many reasons, and I'll highlight a few. It is estimated about one percent of the world's population has Celiac disease (a genetic autoimmune disease and the most severe form of gluten intolerance). While that number is relatively small, it's estimated that thirty to forty percent of people have "non-celiac gluten sensitivity," or NCGS. These people may experience intestinal symptoms (such as bloating, gas, diarrhea, constipation, nausea or abdominal pain) but often they do not. Instead the symptoms of NCGS often include: brain fog, headaches, fatigue, pain, skin rashes, neurologic symptoms, or psychiatric symptoms. Celiac disease can be ruled out with bloodwork, but to see if you have NCGS, a great tool is an elimination diet--simply eliminate gluten completely for four weeks, and then re-introduce it. There is no harm in doing this and it can potentially give you answers to an underlying cause of your most nagging health complaints. During your four weeks of remaining gluten free, take note on how you feel. Key areas to pay attention to are: digestion, skin, mood, and energy. Often my clients see improvements in one or more of these areas. At the end of your four-week trial, re-introduce gluten and take note if any symptoms return. This will give you key information—you can then make an educated choice of whether or not to eat gluten in the future. Choosing to abstain from eating gluten can be empowering, rather than depriving, if it means living with better health and happiness.

Another reason, aside from Celiac disease and gluten-sensitivity, to discontinue eating gluten, is that wheat is sprayed with a chemical weed killer, glyphosate (i.e. Roundup). Glyphosate exposure is linked to leaky gut, cancer, and other illnesses. As humans, we do not need to be eating gluten. There are many other good sources of nutrition without the harmful effects of modern wheat products.

In 2013, my husband and I agreed to remove gluten from our home and our diets. We agreed to do a one-month trial—it seemed impossible, but I had a friend who had done it with positive outcomes. Within three days of removing gluten from our home and our diets, we noticed that our child with rashes (eczema) and poor energy, suddenly was rash-free and had better energy! Within two weeks, I noticed my sleep felt more restorative and I had steady energy all day, instead of the peaks and valleys that had become my norm. My husband, a lifelong allergy sufferer, noticed a marked decrease in his congestion and sneezing. Fast-forward to now, we have chosen as a family to continue to be gluten-free. We feel better this way, and we don't feel deprived. You may already be on board with gluten-free, or you may think it sounds bonkers. After growing up eating cereal, bread, and pasta every day, how could anyone survive without gluten? Honestly, the first few days (for some people, the first two weeks) are difficult because you have to break your addiction (yes, gluten and wheat are addictive) and you have to find new foods/meals to prepare. But I assure you that it gets easier.

Dairy is another common inflammatory food—yes, it contains vitamins and minerals, but it also contains a lot of sugar. A single serving (one cup) of cow milk contains a whopping eleven grams of sugar. I am not anti-dairy, but here's my take: cow milk is the perfect food if you are a baby cow. Just like human breast milk is the perfect food for a baby human. Because we are not baby cows, *we do not need to consume dairy*. I'm not saying it's wrong to consume dairy, but I am saying that it isn't necessary.

Interestingly, I consumed milk and cheese every day of my life up until my thirties. When I did a one-month trial without dairy, I found that my skin cleared up! I had lived with chronic acne since age fifteen. Yes, twenty years of mild to moderate acne—during those years I took many prescription creams and pills, yet I still had acne. But now, without dairy, my skin is clear. If I consume dairy, my acne returns. For this reason, I've chosen to remain dairy-free.

Please note, I am not saying that dairy is the cause of *your* acne (or health issues), but it was for me. I am also not saying that you can never again consume milk, cheese, or yogurt. What I *am* saying is that you need to listen to your body. There is no harm in removing dairy for four weeks and then re-introducing it to see how you feel. Pay attention to your skin, energy, digestion, and mood. Food sensitivities can create symptoms in any or all of these categories. (Note: when I spoke to a conventional dermatologist about my acne/dairy experience, she quickly dismissed me, saying that there was no scientific study to support my experience. First, I think she is incorrect and second, I think it does a disservice to dismiss people when they have found something to be true for them. Each of us knows our bodies and can feel empowered to make decisions based on our own observations.)

If you're a person who can't tolerate dairy, please know that there are other great ways to get your calcium. A few calcium-rich foods include: sesame seeds, sardines, collard greens, spinach, bok choy, and almonds. Some people can tolerate dairy just fine and if that's you, great—choose organic and grass-fed dairy products when possible.

The final inflammatory category is "junk oils." Junk oils are highly processed, industrial seed oils. They are often found in processed foods, frozen foods, salad dressings, and fast foods. These oils are high in omega-6 which increases inflammation in the body, and they are often rancid by the time you purchase them!

Junk oils to avoid:

- Soybean oil
- Canola oil
- Corn oil
- Safflower oil

- Palm oil
- Peanut oil
- Vegetable oil
- Vegetable shortening
- Margarine (and other "fake butters")
- Anything that says "hydrogenated"

In addition to eliminating (or greatly reducing) sugar, processed foods, gluten, dairy and junk oils, I have a few more recommendations to help you reduce sources of inflammation.

The quality of the food you consume is very important. I suggest that you avoid foods with pesticides, antibiotics, hormones, food dyes, chemicals, preservatives, and artificial sweeteners. It's important to reduce the chemical "burden" to your body. Switching to organic foods is worth it in my opinion. The Environmental Working Group (EWG) states, "Organic foods cannot be irradiated; genetically modified; or grown with synthetic pesticides or fertilizers, chemical additives or sewage sludge. Organic livestock and poultry cannot be treated with hormones and antibiotics" ("What does organic mean?, 2017). Unfortunately, if we are not careful, many of these listed toxins are in our food and they have been linked to many of the chronic diseases we face as a nation.

My husband and I have decided to invest in organic food. We agreed that we would rather pay now to protect our health than pay later with illness and medical bills. If you are new to switching from conventional produce to organic produce, the dirty dozen is a good list to follow. These foods are the most "contaminated" and therefore a good place to invest in purchasing organic.

2018 Dirty Dozen: Fruits and Veggies with the Most Pesticides:

(i.e. choose organic whenever possible)

- Strawberries
- Spinach
- Nectarines
- Apples
- Grapes
- Peaches
- Cherries
- Pears
- Tomatoes
- Celery
- Potatoes
- Sweet bell peppers

2018 Clean Fifteen: Fruits and Veggies with the Least Pesticides:

(i.e. considered "safe" to consume conventionally grown)

- Avocados
- Sweet Corn
- Pineapples

- Cabbages
- Onions
- Sweet peas
- Papayas
- Asparagus
- Mangos
- Eggplants
- Honeydews
- Kiwis
- Cantaloupes
- Cauliflower
- Broccoli

That concludes the section of which foods to avoid. Next, here are a few guidelines on how to properly nourish with food.

1. **Eat lots of vegetables.** Choose a variety of vegetables and a variety of colors. Vegetables contain vitamins, minerals, and phytonutrients; all of which help to fight disease and promote health. They are also a great source of fiber. Fiber helps with gut health and proper digestion. A diet high in fibrous vegetables can help you lose weight. For optimal health, aim to eat veggies at every meal. Fill one quarter to half of your plate with non-starchy and colorful veggies. Good options include spinach,

kale, asparagus, broccoli, arugula, brussels sprouts, cabbage, celery, cucumbers, radishes, and artichokes. Note: Nightshades, including bell peppers, eggplant, potatoes, and tomatoes are nutritious options for most people. However, some people have difficulty digesting these, which can lead to bloating and pain. If you have arthritis or autoimmune disease, or you suspect you are allergic to nightshades, remove them from your diet for a few weeks and see how you feel.

2. **Eat high-quality protein.** Choose organic, grass-fed, hormone- and antibiotic-free whenever possible. Keep in mind that protein does not need to be your main course; plant-based foods should take center stage and the animal protein can be more like the side dish. I like the rule that a serving of protein is about the size of your palm. Good sources of protein include: eggs, beef, lamb, chicken, turkey, wild-caught salmon, cod, shrimp, seeds and nuts, and beans and lentils. It's up to you to discover which protein sources work best for your body.

3. **Consume healthy fats and oils.** Despite what you may have been conditioned to believe, fat does *not* make you fat, and eating fat does not cause heart attacks. Dr. Mark Hyman explains the facts and the science behind this in his book, *Food: What the Heck Should I Eat?* (Hyman, 2018, pp.151-154). I

mentioned earlier that some oils are inflammatory, so make sure you keep those in mind as oils to throw away and never purchase again. Now, why do you need to consume healthy fats? They help you feel satiated, they help stabilize blood sugar, and they help increase metabolism. Fats are necessary for healthy cell membranes and for producing hormones.

Healthy fats to consume include:

- Extra virgin olive oil
- Organic coconut oil
- Avocado oil
- Grass-fed butter (if you tolerate dairy)
- Ghee (clarified butter)

When purchasing olive oil, be sure to purchase high quality; it should have a dark green color and taste strongly of olives. Please beware that if it does not meet these criteria, it may be "counterfeit," meaning it will be low quality or will be a nut or soybean oil. Another thing you should know is that olive oil is best used as a drizzle and not for cooking at high heat. When cooking at high heat on the stove or in the oven, I suggest you use coconut oil or avocado oil because they have a higher smoke point. Nuts, seeds, and avocados are also great sources of healthy fats. Nuts to consume include almonds, cashews, walnuts, macadamias, pecans, and brazil. Seeds to consume include pumpkin, flax, sesame, chia, hemp, and sunflower.

4. **Choose starchy foods that are gluten-free.** Choose gluten-free grains like quinoa, oats (must be labeled gluten-free), rice, buckwheat, teff, and amaranth. More good options for plant-based starchy foods include sweet potatoes, winter squash, legumes, and lentils. If you are diabetic or have a weight loss goal, you may want to eat smaller portions of these starchy foods.

5. **Eat fresh, seasonal fruits.** I see fruit as "nature's candy." Once you clean up your diet and nourish with high-quality and nutrient-dense foods, fresh fruit really is quite enjoyable. It's true that fruit contains valuable vitamins, minerals, phytonutrients, and fiber, however one drawback is that fruit contains sugar (in the form of fructose). I suggest one to three servings of fresh fruit per day (one serving equals half a cup). Dried fruit is an okay option but it's best reserved as a treat and in moderation due to the sugar content. Please avoid fruit juice—it's high in sugar and low in nutritional value. Good fruit choices include fresh berries, frozen berries, stone fruit (peaches, plums, nectarines, cherries), melons, apples, pears, bananas, and citrus fruits. If you're overweight, diabetic, or have blood sugar issues, then it's best to stick to low sugar fruits like berries (blueberries, cherries, blackberries, raspberries), apples, and pears.

6. **Add foods that boost gut health.** Bone broth

made from organic bones (such as chicken or beef) contains important minerals and collagen that promote the healing of gut walls. Bone broth can be used as a base for soups and stews, it can be used for cooking rice, or it can be consumed as a beverage. Probiotic and prebiotic foods help to promote the growth of good bacteria in the gut. Probiotic foods include fermented sauerkraut or pickles, kimchi, or kombucha. Aim for two tablespoons per day. Prebiotic foods help feed the good bacteria and these include plant-based foods such as leeks, onions, garlic, asparagus, artichokes, cucumbers, celery, oatmeal, beans, berries, apples, pears, nuts, and flaxseeds.

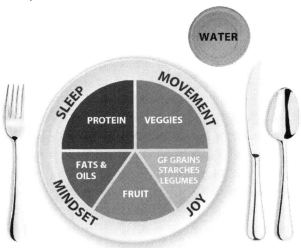

Ready, Set, Heal

These guidelines work great for most people; however, there's flexibility within this plan. One person may thrive on animal protein, while another thrives on vegetarian protein. Some of my clients thrive with very little to no grains. Some thrive with moderate amounts of grains. You are unique and it's important to listen to your body and intuition to guide which foods work best for you. When I work one on one with my clients, I help them figure out which foods work well and which foods don't work well for them.

Food allergies and food sensitivities are on the rise among children *and* adults. You may already know what foods you're allergic to or sensitive to. Many of my clients do. They say things like, "I get a stomach ache if I have too much milk or cheese," or, "my skin gets itchy if I eat too much gluten," or, "I have trouble sleeping if I drink coffee after one p.m." Some confess things like, "I feel anxious after I eat a lot of sugar," and, "dairy gives me loose stools."

If you monitor your energy, moods, skin, and bowel habits, you will gain a lot of information as to which foods you are sensitive to. Listen to these clues! Often once my clients eliminate their allergenic foods, they begin to see significant positive changes within two to four weeks. One of my clients noticed that sugar caused digestive distress—once she committed to removing sugar from her diet, she lost twenty pounds with ease! Additionally, she gained confidence, improved moods, improved productivity with her work, and more satisfaction with her life as a busy mom.

Another tip to help you properly nourish with food is to slow down when you eat. Eating is meant to happen in a state of relaxation. When we're rushing, we're in a state of fight-or-flight—and the body shunts blood away from digestive organs when stress is high. I encourage you to take a few deep breaths before you start eating. Take a moment to observe the high-quality food you are about to nourish with. Notice the colors and the smells. This mindfulness will prep your brain to release digestive enzymes and gastric juices to prepare for the incoming foods. Be grateful for the farmer. Have gratitude that you (or your family member) took time to plan that meal, shop for that meal, and prepare that meal. Remember to fully chew your food. Taste the flavors, notice the textures. Chew fully—to the consistency of baby food—before you swallow. Your stomach does not have teeth. Undigested food is wasted food. You want your body to be able to extract as many vitamins and minerals as it can from your food.

As you begin nourishing with more high-quality foods, you'll likely feel more energized and satisfied. Your bloating will disappear and you'll likely shed excess weight with ease. You will experience firsthand what people mean when they say, "Nothing tastes as good as being healthy feels." You get to choose how to nourish yourself and therefore it shouldn't feel depriving. Instead, I hope you feel empowered and grateful for the healthy choices you're making. Eating is meant to be satisfying, so please slow down and enjoy it!

Nourish with food action steps:

1. Clean out your fridge and pantry. Get rid of processed foods with artificial colors, high fructose corn syrup, and long or cryptic ingredient lists. Get rid of inflammatory oils (see list above). If you plan to do a gluten and/or dairy-free trial, remove those foods from your home.

2. Re-stock your fridge and pantry with the healthy oils and other foods suggested above.

3. Eat vegetables at every meal. (For example, have leftover veggies with your eggs for breakfast, eat a big salad for lunch, and include lots of vegetables with dinner).

4. Switch from conventional to organic produce (especially the dirty dozen list).

5. When consuming animal protein, choose high-quality grass-fed or pasture-raised meats—healthy animals produce healthy meat (more nutrients, less antibiotics, and so on). Remember that a portion is the size of your palm.

6. Consume healthy fats. Good choices include extra virgin olive oil, organic coconut oil, avocados, nuts, and seeds.

7. Enjoy gluten-free grains and starchy foods like squash, legumes, and lentils.

8. Enjoy fresh, seasonal organic fruit in moderation. It

truly is nature's candy.

9. Add gut-health promoting foods like bone broth and fermented foods.

10. Prepare a meal plan for your week and let that guide your grocery shopping. Keep the meals simple. Cook once, eat twice; this means if you cook one meal, you can enjoy it two nights in a row, or have it for dinner one night and then lunch the next day.

11. Do more home cooking and less eating out. You'll be more in control of the quality of foods and the portion sizes when you prepare them.

12. Slow down, relax, and fully chew your food. Eating is meant to be enjoyable.

13. Follow the 80:20 rule. Eighty percent of the time follow the above rules. Release the need to be one hundred percent perfect with food choices, as this often creates unnecessary stress. Of course, if you have a food sensitivity or allergy, it's best to avoid that food one hundred percent.

NOURISH WITH WATER

"The body's solution to pollution is dilution."

-Unknown

You've likely heard that your body is made up of sixty to seventy-five percent water. So, it should be no surprise that how much (or how little) you drink can affect your health. Too much water can result in mineral imbalances, while too little can cause dehydration, headaches, muscle stiffness, and fatigue. Additionally, water helps with detoxification. We live in a world full of toxins—toxins in the air we breathe, in the self-care products we smear on our skin (our largest organ; unfortunately, it absorbs a lot), and in our food (pesticides and herbicides) if it isn't organic. Drinking sufficient amounts of clean water will help you clear these toxins from your body as well as have clearer skin, improved elimination, and improved appetite control. You've probably noticed that when you're dehydrated, you're often hungrier. The brain has a hard time differentiating between thirst and hunger.

How much water should you drink each day? A general rule of thumb is to drink half your body weight in ounces of water. For example, someone who weighs one hundred forty pounds needs to drink approximately seventy ounces of water per day. Since there are eight ounces per cup, that equates to eight and a half cups of water per day. So, if this person uses a twenty-four-ounce water bottle, they'll need to drink three full water bottles per day. This isn't an exact science and you must listen to your body to find the amount of water that best suits you each day. Keep in mind that during the summer, after exercise, or during pregnancy, you may require additional water.

Let's talk about water bottles. I think reusable water bottles are great, but I urge you to use stainless-steel or glass. Reusable plastic water bottles are not ideal (yes, even the PBA-free ones) because the plastics can leech into your water and then you'll be drinking contaminated water. Plastic in the body is a hormone disrupter. Hormone disrupters (also called endocrine disrupters) are chemicals that interfere with the body's hormonal signaling. It's best to avoid these chemicals because they've been linked to cancers, fertility issues, and more. Please get a new water bottle if you need to. This will be twenty dollars well spent.

Do you drink bottled spring water? Even though it is marketed to you as being "from a mountain spring," it comes in a thin plastic bottle. Those bottles sit on pallets in hot trucks as they're transported from a factory to a store. The heat causes additional leeching of plastic into the water. We don't yet know all the long-term effects of these chemicals, but with the rates of hormonal imbalances, infertility, and cancers skyrocketing, it's not worth the risk for me. It can be difficult to avoid disposable plastic water bottles at social events and while traveling, but in your daily routine, you can eliminate them.

Are you drinking tap water? Unfortunately, your tap water may contain unwanted contaminates like arsenic, lead, mercury, chromium-6, chlorine, and more. Water filters are a worthwhile investment. There are many great options and here are a few to consider.

1. Big Berkey Water Filter System (I have this)

2. New Wave Enviro 10 stage countertop water filtration system

3. Aquasana Water Filter System

4. Reverse osmosis whole house water filtration system (a bigger investment; one I plan to make in the future)

Bonus Tip: When possible, drink water between meals rather than during meals. The stomach is highly acidic (pH 1.4) for proper breakdown and digestion of food. Water is neutral (pH 7), and can alter that acidic environment.

How do I get my proper intake of water each day? I start my day with one to two cups of herbal tea or water. I then sip water throughout the day, refilling my reusable stainless-steel water bottle as needed. I take this water bottle with me anytime I leave the house, even when traveling.

Nourish with water action steps:

1. Drink seven to nine cups of water per day (approximately half your body weight in ounces).

2. Drink water from a reusable glass or stainless-steel water bottle.

3. Drink one to two cups of water first thing in the morning—as soon as you wake up.

4. Drink most of your water between meals; limit water intake during your meal.

5. Invest in a water filtration system (see ideas above).

NOURISH WITH SLEEP

Do you wake up fully refreshed and full of energy each morning? Or are you like so many women who wake up feeling groggy and wish they could pull the covers back over their heads? Maybe you avoid getting out of bed because the tasks of the day and the stressors in your life feel overwhelming. Or maybe you drag yourself out of bed knowing that coffee is around the corner and it'll give you the jumpstart you need to get your brain and body moving. Whatever your unique scenario is, I can almost guarantee that you're not alone. We're a nation of sleep-deprived individuals. We have become accustomed to believe that notion, "I'll sleep when I'm dead." We're trained to go, go, go, and then go some more. But we aren't machines. We're human beings—we're mammals! Sometimes we forget this. Does your dog or cat "go" with endless energy all day? Probably not. They have periods of high activity and periods of rest each day. And they most certainly sleep—a lot! Maybe they know something we've forgotten?

How do you feel when you're sleep deprived? If you're like me and my clients, you likely experience increased cravings, your thinking is impaired, and you feel irritable and short-tempered. Sleep deprivation often leads to a vicious cycle of sugar cravings and energy crashes. Additionally, chronic sleep deprivation will lower your immune system. This is *not* helpful if you're trying to lose weight and feel great. And what busy woman (or mom) has time for slowed thinking or getting sick? I don't! My kids are smart and they keep me on my toes--I need to think fast *and* I need to avoid illness to keep up with them.

Proper sleep is essential for optimal health and happiness. During sleep, the body repairs and restores itself. How amazing is that? Your body is designed to heal—and sleep is when it does some of its best healing. During sleep, your tissues rebuild and toxins are eliminated. Plus, your brain consolidates the experiences from the day and organizes it into new knowledge. In her book *The Adrenal Thyroid Revolution,* Dr. Aviva Romm says that, "Sleep is the ultimate pause button you need at the end of the day," and, "You need at least seven hours of good sleep every night to reset your natural clock and cortisol rhythm, to dump the chemical toxins that accumulate in your brain and body all day, and for your brain to do the work of sorting and filing new information from that day"(Romm, p.177).

How much sleep do you need? Most women require seven to nine hours. When I was recovering from my health crash in 2014, I needed nine to ten hours per night. Currently, I find that I feel best with eight hours. What amount of sleep is your sweet spot? Be honest with yourself.

If you're having difficulty sleeping, there are many steps you can take to improve your sleep, naturally. As a mammal, you're designed to be awake when the sun is up and sleep when the sun is down. Optimizing the quality and quantity of your sleep will provide you many health benefits. Look at this list and see what you're doing well, and where you can make improvements.

Lauren's top tips for optimizing sleep:

- Routine is key—go to bed and wake up at same time every day.

- Get sun exposure first thing in the morning. Sit by a window while you eat breakfast or get outside for a short walk (or other exercise).

- Exercise at least thirty minutes per day (preferably not within two hours of bedtime)

- Avoid coffee and other forms of caffeine after one p.m. (including chocolate if you are highly sensitive to caffeine).

- Watch the sunset when possible. This helps with resetting cortisol and melatonin, which are important hormones for your sleep-wake cycle.

- Reduce or eliminate overhead lighting in the evenings; overhead lighting confuses your brain to make you think it's high noon all day long.

- Turn on "nightshift" if you have an iPhone (or download Twilight for Android) to reduce blue light. Blue light affects circadian rhythms. Set nightshift mode to turn on from seven p.m. to seven a.m.

- End screen time one hour before bed; try reading in bed with a dim light or listen to an audiobook or guided meditation to relax before sleep.

- Establish a bedtime routine for you, just like you have a routine for your kids.

- While sleeping, set phone on airplane mode or better yet, turn it off to reduce EMF (electromagnetic field) exposure. We don't yet know the long-term effects of EMF.

- Turn off Wi-Fi in the house while sleeping by plugging the router into an outlet timer. Some studies show that Wi-Fi negatively affects circadian rhythm and sleep. An outlet timer can be purchased at your local home improvement store or from Amazon for less than fifteen dollars. My husband was reluctant to make this change, but once we did, we noticed an improvement in our children's health and behavior. Happy kids means happy parents! Our timer is set to turn off Wi-Fi every night from ten p.m. to six a.m.

- Bedrooms should be tidy, free of clutter, and very dark (blackout curtains). Your bedroom should be reserved for sleep and intimacy only; remove the television, exercise equipment, work materials, and clutter.

If the above steps are not enough...

- Diffuse lavender essential oil one hour before bed

- Drink a soothing bedtime tea with chamomile or lavender

- Perform deep breathing (4-7-8 technique)—view this video by Dr. Andrew Weil (https://www.drweil.com/videos-features/videos/breathing-exercises-4-7-8-breath/)

- Try magnesium supplementation, also known as the "relaxation mineral." One suggestion is *Natural Calm* powder (magnesium citrate). Alternatively, you could take an evening bath with Epsom salt (magnesium sulfate).

Key questions to consider:

- How do you feel when you're sleep deprived?

- How do you feel when you get several nights of great sleep?

- What are your health goals?

- Do you believe that better sleep will contribute to you reaching your goals?

Nourish with sleep action steps:

1. Make sleep a priority.

2. Write down how many hours of sleep you need to feel your best. _____

3. Write down what time you plan to wake up each day. _____

4. Write down what time you plan to go sleep. _____

5. Read the list of tips for improving your sleep. Note which areas you would like to work on with an asterisk.

NOURISH WITH MOVEMENT

"Take care of your body, it's the only place you have to live."

-Jim Rohn

Are you exercising at least thirty minutes, five days per week? If yes, I commend you. If no, you're not alone. In this chapter, I'll share my views and recommendations when it comes to moving our bodies in ways that nourish us. But before I get to my recommendations on this topic, I want to address some issues that many women experience related to exercise.

Have you ever signed up for a gym membership and you go diligently for the first few weeks, only to "fall off the wagon" and stop going? You know you should be going, you know you're paying a monthly membership, yet you still don't go and you feel bad about yourself. Feeling guilt or shame about your lack of exercise doesn't make the situation any better—in fact, it causes additional stress chemicals (cortisol) to be released in your body. Many people pay for gym memberships they don't use and everyone I know struggles with some amount of negative self-talk. It's my hope that this chapter helps you find some peace around the topic of exercise and helps you take baby steps in implementing an exercise routine you feel good about.

There's a reason I titled this chapter "Nourish with Movement" rather than "Nourish with Exercise." I've learned that many women have a negative association with the idea of "exercise." Often this negative association starts in childhood—maybe you were the last one picked for a team in gym class, or maybe you weren't an athlete, maybe you got teased for your athletic abilities, or maybe you never enjoyed sports and never discovered alternate ways to exercise that you did enjoy.

One client I worked with really wanted to incorporate exercise into her weekly routine, yet each time we met, she again had neglected to do the exercise routine we'd discussed. As a heath coach, it's not my position to judge. Instead, I get curious as to why the plan isn't being implemented.

Upon discussion, this woman realized that she *hates* exercise! She didn't consciously realize this until we really got talking. It turned out that just the thought of exercise brought up many negative emotions—shame, embarrassment, discomfort, and more. She traced her negative association to "exercise" back to middle and high school gym class. On her gym days she got sweaty, her hair got messy, and then the rest of the school day she felt embarrassed and dirty. Additionally, the exercises she was forced to do were not what she enjoyed, nor did she feel adept when doing them. On her non-gym days, she felt prettier and more confident. The negative emotions that she tied to exercise stayed with her well into adulthood!

Once she realized this, we stopped using the word "exercise" and instead began using the word "movement." From there, we discussed ways that she enjoys moving her body. She revealed that she loves to do Qui Gong in her backyard. In the end, this was the movement we added to her routine and it worked for her.

There is no "one size fits all" approach to exercise. There are important principles, but there is variation from one person to the next. Sure, as a physical therapist, I think it would be ideal for all people to do cardiovascular exercise, core and functional strength training, and stretching. These three types of movement each serve a unique purpose in keeping our physical body healthy. But each person is unique and each person has to find a routine that works for them. A marathon runner will have a much different routine from someone who has been sedentary for several years.

If you have a physical injury or movement limitation, I encourage you to see a physical therapist. A physical therapist can help you restore your movement and can help you design an exercise program that's safe for you. A proper exercise program can help you build strength, endurance, balance, and confidence. If you struggle with chronic pain, a physical therapist can help you design a program to get you started. It may sound daunting, but being sedentary is not helpful; rather, it's detrimental for those with chronic pain.

If you don't have an injury or movement limitation, then I encourage you to think about what types of movement or exercise you enjoy. If you enjoy it and feel good about it, then you are much more likely to build it into your routine and stick with it. The perfect routine is the one that works for you.

Let's review the benefits to exercise and then we can move into finding exercise or movement that works for you. The benefits to exercise are many. Many of my clients struggle with low energy and a sluggish metabolism. Exercise helps with these things and so much more. In addition to a healthy diet, it's one of the best tools for improving your health and happiness. As you read this list, please think about which benefits appeal to you.

Benefits of exercise:
- Weight management
- Improves mood
- Reduces inflammation
- Improves digestion
- Improves quality of sleep
- Improves strength
- Improves balance
- Improves flexibility
- Improves bone density
- Reduces joint and back pain
- Improves heart health
- Improves blood pressure
- Improves immune function
- Improves liver health

- Improves insulin sensitivity
- Improves cognitive function
- Improves energy

If you're sedentary or have not exercised consistently for a while, then I recommend you begin with a walking program. The body is designed to walk! We start walking around the age of one and we continue to walk throughout our lifetime. Some people might believe that walking doesn't count as exercise, but this simply isn't true. Many of my clients have successfully improved their health and happiness during my coaching program by adding walking. Brisk walking from thirty to sixty minutes, five days per week, is where my clients see the greatest benefit in improved energy, improved mood, and weight loss. You may need to start with ten minutes, and that's okay too. Start somewhere.

While walking is great, you may have other forms of movement that you enjoy. As I mentioned, if you choose something you enjoy, you're much more likely to stick with it. If it feels like a chore, then it will likely not last. As women, we're already busy, so the last thing we need is to add one more chore to our list, right?

What forms of movement do you enjoy?
- Walking
- Yoga
- Pilates
- Tai chi

- Spin classes
- Cycling
- Swimming
- Running
- Dancing
- Hiking
- Recreational sports (volleyball, softball, soccer, etc.)

Do you prefer to exercise alone or with other people? Exercising alone helps some women feel like they are recharging their battery. But other women prefer to exercise with a friend for that added accountability—which I like to call a "social contract." And other women prefer to exercise in groups because they feed off the energy of the group. Do you prefer to exercise indoors or outdoors? Answering these questions will help you gain clarity about what's best for you. Personally, I enjoy the positive energy in group classes, but I also really love to be outdoors whenever possible. I try to jog two or three days per week followed by a few minutes of stretching. I also do five minutes of yoga in my backyard several days each week. If time permits, I try to get to one group exercise class per week.

Maybe jogging and yoga aren't your thing, and you instead love to dance. But you're a mom and you work full time, so taking a dance class would add to your already full schedule. Maybe you can turn on some music and dance around with your kids a few evenings each week? And you can take a walk during your lunch break for ten to twenty minutes per day. Get creative and think about what you enjoy and where you can build it into your routine. These small pieces of exercise will add up. You will likely feel stronger and more energized.

I can't leave the topic of movement and exercise without addressing something I see all too often. Many women use exercise as a means of "burning calories" and/or punishment. After indulging in sweets or overeating, you might find yourself thinking, "I better go exercise to burn this off." Our society has taught us women to think this way, but it's a very unhealthy pattern. I know, because I was there. During the peak of the low-fat era (which happened to be when I was in college), I was addicted to carbs and sugar. My energy was low and I was constantly craving sugar for that instant hit of energy. I gained weight, and the freshman fifteen became the sophomore thirty.

During college, I hit my peak weight (aside from pregnancy) and I was thirty pounds heavier than I am today. I felt uncomfortable in my body and I believed that if I could just lose the weight, I'd be happy. After eating sweets (or even binging), I punished myself with hard workouts, and then when I didn't lose weight, I gave up. This became a cycle and I never did lose the weight with this method.

It wasn't until I formed a healthier relationship with food, exercise, and myself, that the weight came off with ease. It takes time to overcome these negative patterns, but it is possible. Be patient with yourself. Focus on nourishment with quality food, movement you enjoy, and the other topics in this book. Experience for yourself what can happen. It requires consistent effort to change your thoughts and habits, but it's a whole lot more fun than torturing yourself with deprivation of calories and punishing with over-exercising. Try to shift your mindset to view exercise as another way to nourish your body.

One of my clients, Kerri, was stuck in a pattern of exercising to "burn calories" for over two decades. During her health coaching program with me, she shifted to viewing food as nourishment and exercise as nourishment. She found a way of eating that left her feeling satisfied and empowered. And she began to exercise for the immediate benefits of feeling strong, feeling a boost in her mood, and feeling a boost in her energy. She now loves doing at-home DVD workouts six days per week.

Nourish with Movement questions to consider:

1. What are your favorite forms of movement or exercise?

2. Do you prefer to exercise alone or with others?

3. Do you prefer to exercise indoors or outdoors?

4. How do you feel during and after exercise?

5. Review the Benefits of Exercise list above. Circle each benefit that appeals to you.

6. Schedule exercise into your week. Start with a very small, achievable goal and build gradually.

NOURISH WITH MINDSET

"The body achieves what the mind believes"

-Anonymous

Foster Hope: If you had shared the above quote with me five years ago, I would've dismissed it. Or if I really thought about it, I would have called it B.S. I mean, I knew that my hard work paid off so I could get good grades, excel in sports, etc., but ultimately, I felt like my destiny wasn't really in my control. I felt like a lot of success in life came down to luck, or fate, or whatever.

But my belief system has shifted. I now believe that the majority of my outcomes depend on my thoughts and actions. Of course, some things are beyond my control and sometimes unlucky (or unfortunate) things happen. But more often than not, my life experiences are a result of my thoughts, my actions, and my reactions.

My observations throughout my career, my own health recovery, the recovery of my colleagues who are health coaches and functional medicine doctors, and numerous books I have read on the subject have all taught me the same thing—in order to reclaim your health and happiness, you must first believe that you can. That is worth repeating—in order to heal, you must first believe that healing is possible. I had to believe that healing was possible, or how would I have found the motivation to follow my daily self-prescription? Without belief and hope, your chances of achieving anything diminish. And what is the harm in having hope?

How can you foster hope? One way is to remember that your body is an amazing biocomputer that is programmed to heal. Your body is far more capable of healing than you have been led to believe. And the more you nourish it in the ways I describe in this book, the more it will do what it is so brilliantly designed to do.

Focus on success. The brain is like a GPS system. What we think about, we bring about. Here's a short story to illustrate when I first learned this lesson. I was twenty-three when I went mountain biking for the first time with some friends. I was living in Maryland and there are some great trails—many of which are single track, meaning a very narrow trail. My friends specifically told me, "When we get to the narrow part of the trail with the steep cliff on one side, whatever you do, focus on the trail and *do not look down.*" They were very clear with this instruction.

However, when we got to the narrow part of the trail, I got scared. And you know what I did? I looked down! And where do you think I went? That's right, I went head over handlebars down the cliff. I reached to grab whatever I could to slow down—which unfortunately were pricker bushes! Thankfully, aside from many scratches, I was fine. But the lesson stayed with me—*where you look is where you go.* So, please, in every aspect of your life, your health, your relationships, and your career—focus on where you want to go.

Early in my healing journey, my therapist confided in me that she'd had a similar health crash several years earlier. Fortunately, she was able to put her pieces back together. She had returned to a productive and happy life—she felt good about her parenting, her relationships, and her career. If she could do it, then I hoped that I could too. For your situation, you may know people who have been through similar challenges. I encourage you to look for success stories. Look for stories of hope. Put blinders on. Stop looking where you don't want to go. The success stories may offer you important clues, lessons, or hope. Create an image of what success looks like for you and focus on that.

Stress Less. If I told you to relax more and stress less, you intuitively would know that these are good for your health, but they're easier said than done, right? Let's talk about the stress response system in the body. If you took biology or anatomy and physiology, you may have learned about the Autonomic Nervous System (ANS). The ANS is the part of your nervous system (brain and body) that controls your automatic bodily functions. The ANS controls breathing, digestion, maintaining homeostasis of temperature, blood pressure, and many more functions.

The ANS has two parts—the sympathetic and the

parasympathetic nervous system. You're already familiar with the sympathetic nervous system—you call it "fight or flight." It's that moment you're with your kids in a crowded place and you suddenly can't find your child. He was just there a few seconds ago! You start looking around, your heart starts racing, your pupils dilate, and you're on high alert. Phew, there he is! You found him, and now you take a few deep breaths and your heart rate starts to return to normal. The sympathetic nervous system is a survival mechanism. In emergency situations, it activates to allow you to do just that—fight or flee a dangerous situation.

Historically, this sympathetic nervous system response activated in emergency situations (like running from a tiger), but otherwise the body returned to a resting state controlled by the parasympathetic nervous system. This relaxed state allows the body to rest, digest, and heal. In nature, constant stress is rare. But unfortunately, our modern lifestyle is characterized by constant stress. The body can either be in a sympathetic or parasympathetic state at any given moment, but not both at the same time. So, if you're in a constant (or near constant) state of stress, then your body is predominately in a sympathetic state. This bathes your cells in stress hormones and can trigger inflammation. It is my goal for you to learn how to spend more time in a relaxed, or parasympathetic state, because that's when your body will be able to rest, digest, and heal.

How can you turn off the stress response and allow for activation of the parasympathetic nervous system? Everyone has stress; this is normal. But there are healthy ways to manage or even lessen the stress response. Deep breathing is one option with great benefits and little to no risk.

4-7-8 breathing is a technique made famous by Dr. Andrew Weil, a pioneer in integrative medicine. It is powerful because once you learn it, you can shift out of sympathetic and into parasympathetic in a matter of seconds. Visit this web address to view a video of Dr. Weil teaching this.

https://www.drweil.com/videos-features/videos/breathing-exercises-4-7-8-breath/

Here's how to do the technique: Start by sitting or lying in a comfortable position. Then, place the tip of your tongue against the ridge of tissue just behind your upper front teeth and keep it there during this exercise; you'll be exhaling through your mouth around your tongue; you may need to purse your lips as well. Here are the steps:

1. Exhale completely through your mouth, making a whoosh sound.

2. Close your mouth and inhale quietly through your nose to a mental count of four.

3. Hold your breath for a count of seven.

4. Exhale completely through your mouth, making a whoosh sound to a count of eight. This is one breath cycle.

5. Now inhale again and repeat the cycle three more times for a total of four.

This breathing technique is most effective when you do it two times a day. It takes practice, but you'll know when you master it because you'll feel an immediate relaxation in your body. Note: if 4-7-8 breathing feels complicated, you can start with a simpler technique of "smell the roses, pause, then blow out the candles" with a focus on your exhale being twice as long as your inhale. Repeat for a total of four breaths.

Release perfectionism. Many of the women I work with consider themselves perfectionists. The have very high standards for themselves and when they don't meet them, they feel like they're failing. If they set out to exercise three times per week but only exercise twice, they often feel bad about it. But I see it differently. Each small win is still a win. This often happens in the area of nutrition too. They feel like they need to follow the nutrition plan one hundred percent or they fail. But eating well eighty percent of the time is amazing! This provides the body with so many important vitamins and minerals. In most cases, a few sweet treats don't negate all the good nourishment.

Perfectionism adds extra stress. It can feel defeating. It can stop us from doing things because of the fear of doing them imperfectly. I've had perfectionist tendencies most of my life and I've worked hard to overcome them. I no longer consider myself a perfectionist; instead I refer to myself as a "high achiever." The following two mantras have helped me and I hope they can be of help to you.

"Done is better than perfect"

and

"good enough is good enough."

Overcome Limiting Beliefs. What are limiting beliefs? These are any beliefs or statements about yourself that you believe to be solid truth, yet they may not be. Limiting beliefs are often negative thoughts and they keep you from achieving your goals. So, if you hear yourself saying, "I will always suffer from my autoimmune disease symptoms," replace that statement with, "I am doing what I need to do to improve my health." Or if you say, "I'm never going to lose the weight," replace it with, "I'm nourishing my body with healthy foods, exercise that feels good, and I'm bringing more joy into my life so I can shed the weight and feel great!"

Limiting beliefs can be overcome. The first step is to identify them. The second step is to re-write the script. Anytime you hear negative thoughts enter your mind, replace them with the positive ones. You may notice that your negative thoughts are rooted in fear. It takes time and practice, but limiting beliefs can be overcome. You *can* do this.

Practice forgiveness. Everyone has been hurt. Everyone has emotional pain. I encourage you to forgive yourself for your past and I encourage you to forgive others. This doesn't mean you'll forget. Forgiveness allows us to lighten the emotional load we carry—the emotional weight which can trigger thoughts of anger, resentment, stress, and depression. I like this quote:

"Forgive others, not because they deserve forgiveness, but because you deserve peace."

-Jonathan Lockwood Huie

Note: There are many great therapists who can help you with forgiveness if you're struggling in this area.

Create a gratitude practice. One of my favorite aphorisms is, "It is not grateful people who are happy, but happy people who are grateful." Do you agree? Do you have a gratitude practice? Starting a gratitude practice has been a game changer in my health and happiness. I'll be honest, I had to force myself to do it initially, and it felt uncomfortable. Over time, it has become woven into my daily way of thinking and being. I feel so much gratitude for my health, my kids, my husband, my comfy bed, my silly cats, my clients, and the list goes on. I made this shift with a simple tool--a gratitude journal. I write in a journal daily and I encourage my health coaching clients to do the same.

There is always something to be grateful for. There will always be a mix of good and bad things in your life and in the world at large. So much of how we experience life is a matter of our perception and our perspective.

"We can complain because rose bushes have thorns or rejoice because thorn bushes have roses."

-Abraham Lincoln

Nourish with mindset action steps:

1. Do you have hope that you can improve your health and happiness?

2. Describe what better health looks and feels like for you. Visualize this daily.

3. Try 4-7-8 breathing to lower stress levels and activate the relaxation response.

4. Release perfectionism. Practice the mantras, "good enough is good enough" and "done is better than perfect".

5. Forgive yourself and others. Seek help from a therapist if needed.

6. Start a gratitude practice. Purchase a small journal to keep next to your bed. Every morning upon waking, write three things you are grateful for (big or small). And every evening, write three things that went well that day. Do this for one week and you will begin to see a shift—do this for one month or more and you will begin to change your thought patterns and form the habit of gratitude. Remember, happy people practice gratitude.

If you want more evidence and inspiration for the impact of mindset on healing, I urge you to read the book *Mind Over Medicine* by Dr. Lissa Rankin.

NOURISH WITH JOY

"Find joy in the ordinary."

-Max Lucado

What is joy? I would describe joy as a feeling of pleasure. Joy is like a little spark of happiness or a spark of gratitude that one can experience several times throughout each day. Based on this definition, what brings you joy? What are the top three things that come to mind? Is it your child's laughter, your dog's unconditional love, is it spending time in your garden? Each of us have unique things that bring us joy.

I will admit that I lost sight of joy when I was stuck in a state of "busy." Those years that I was "go go go," working my fast-paced job as a physical therapist and then coming home to start my second shift as a mom and housewife. It felt like I could hardly catch my breath. I honestly stopped thinking about my needs and what brought me joy because I was putting the needs of my family and the demands of my job first. Maybe you can relate?

Joy was almost a non-existent word in my vocabulary. I'm not a curmudgeon, but it just wasn't a word I used very often. That changed when I read Marie Kondo's books, *Spark Joy* and *The Life-Changing Magic of Tidying Up*. Have you read either of those? Kondo is an organizational expert and *New York Times* best-selling author. From her I learned that each item I own has the ability to bring me joy or detract from it. I literally went through my house and organized and de-cluttered *everything!* I only kept things that I needed and/or brought me joy. It felt silly at first holding up a shirt and asking, "Does this bring me joy"? Or asking the same question while holding a book that I had good intentions of reading for the past decade but never seemed to get around to.

As I ran through Kondo's exercise, things clicked and it got easier with practice. I donated many usable items that no longer brought me joy—that shirt that hung in my closet but I never felt great wearing, all those books I had good intentions of reading, etc. As I released these items, I felt lighter. My life felt more organized and simpler in a way that I craved. I learned which material items brought me joy and which did not. From there, I gained insight as to which relationships brought me joy and which ones I needed better boundaries with. I learned which activities and experiences brought me joy.

One huge breakthrough was that I gained major clarity about my next step in my life—I needed to pursue health coaching so that I could help other women heal through holistic means as I had done. Attending The Institute for Integrative Nutrition was one of the most joyful years of my life. Learning to fill my life with joy seems to put me in the flow of the Universe and I am finding that doors are opening with ease.

As it did with me, learning what brings you joy can take time to sort out. Many of my health coaching clients have difficulty identifying what brings them joy. If this is you, please be patient. Pause for a moment and consider what brought you joy as a child. Was it your beloved pet? Was it a special friendship? Or maybe it was an activity like swimming or gymnastics or horseback riding? Whatever it was, think about it. Enjoy those memories. Also consider any unique qualities and talents that you possess. From these things that once brought you joy, are there ways to incorporate them into your life now? Remember to keep it simple.

Here are a few examples. One of my clients is a highly driven and successful career woman. She was able to infuse joy into her life by making sure to get down on the floor each evening and pet her cats. She also loves eating home-cooked meals with her significant other. She takes gratitude for each of these meals. These were simple ways for her to infuse joy into each day.

Another client loves to have quality time with her kids, she loves horseback riding, and she loves dancing. Incorporating these things into her weekly routine has had positive effects on her health and happiness.

Another client loved to play hockey and listen to country music before becoming a mom. In order to infuse more joy in her life, she signed up for an adult hockey league. Now she enjoys playing roller hockey once a week and listening to country music on her drives!

The important thing here is for you to self-reflect and find simple ways to incorporate more joy into your daily or weekly routine. The things that bring you the most joy tend to be in alignment with your purpose.

What is your purpose? And what do I even mean by "purpose"? If you're religious or spiritual, you likely believe that you are in this life for reason. But maybe the idea of having a purpose is new to you.

I believe that each person is born with a unique life purpose. Discovering and honoring a unique purpose takes time and effort. Successful people take the time to discover their purpose and they pursue it with passion.

I have a deep inner knowing that my purpose is, and always has been, to be a healer. Since childhood I was fascinated with the ability of my body to heal from cuts, muscle strains, and broken bones. When I learned about physical therapy at a career day in seventh grade, it was a lightbulb moment for me. This career was fulfilling in many ways; however, now that I'm a health coach, I feel even more in alignment with my purpose. I feel called to support women, especially moms. I love to inspire and support my clients in their healing journeys. And now, with writing this book, I hope to make an even bigger positive impact on the world.

My purpose guides the choices I make in my life. I realize that I'm fortunate to have discovered and aligned with my purpose. I'm hopeful that you can gain clarity by answering the following questions.

- What are your unique skills?

- What are you passionate about?

- What are some of the experiences in your life that have brought you the most satisfaction? Or the greatest pain?

The answers to these questions may start to point you toward your purpose. If you're still unclear, that's okay too. There are books and YouTube videos devoted to the topic of finding your purpose—a few people who offer great material on this topic include Jonathan Fields, Jack Canfield, and Mastin Kipp.

Once you discover your unique life purpose, you do not need to overhaul your life, but you can start to take baby steps to align with your purpose. One of my clients identified that her purpose is *to spread God's love and kindness*. After some self-reflection, she realized that some of the things that bring her the greatest joy include singing in her church choir, socializing, playing with her children, and volunteering. Each of these activities allow her to spread God's love and kindness. And, by following the principles I taught her (and describe in this book), she enhanced her health and wellness. Good health has become a vehicle for her to better serve her life purpose.

Most of the women I work with have a desire to serve others, but each in a unique way. Most of my clients fall into one of four categories: moms, health care providers, entrepreneurs, and high-achieving career women. They are all in service to others. They all have unique gifts. Most of them know their purpose if they take the time to really think about it. The problem I often see is that they forget (or neglect) to "serve" themselves.

Here's an analogy I like for this situation: imagine you have a cup of water and you keep pouring from it to share with others. Eventually, the cup runs out of water. What if instead, you keep filling your cup and it's overflowing—you can now share the overflow without ever depleting your cup. If the cup is you and the water is your energy and resources, I want you to take care of your needs so that you can serve from a place of overflow. This may sound impossible right now—and that's okay. But keep this analogy in mind. Keep filling your cup—nourish with food, water, movement, mindset, and joy. And eventually, you'll keep your cup full and serve from the overflow. It *is* possible. I try to serve my children and my clients from this overflow. I am human and sometimes my water level lowers—I usually get those old feelings of overwhelm or irritability as my water level lowers, and that's when I know I need to dial in my self-care.

Nourish with joy action steps. Answer these questions:

1. What are three to six things that bring you joy?

2. How can you infuse some of these things into your daily or weekly routine?

3. If you had to guess your purpose, what would you guess it is? It's okay to have more than one.

A SPECIAL SECTION FOR MOMS

Motherhood is amazing and beautiful and *challenging*. Never have I been pushed to my physical and emotional limits like I have since becoming a mom. On top of the obvious demands, many of us are raising children who also have chronic health issues or special needs. Childhood chronic health conditions are on the rise. It is quite possible that your child has a diagnosis of food allergies, anxiety, ADHD, asthma, or autism. I'm going share three topics that come up frequently for the moms that I coach: mom guilt, parenting challenges, and mom intuition.

Mom guilt. You know what I'm talking about. There are things you would like to do for yourself, but you hesitate. You put yourself last--always. You prioritize your kids' needs before your own. At the end of the day, there's no time for you. At the end of the week, you're depleted. You like the suggestions in this book, but just thinking about them activates stress and guilt for you. Going to a group fitness class with other women sounds like a great idea—but it costs money and it takes time away from your kids. That leaves you feeling guilt you just can't escape. Or maybe you've been craving a professional massage because the one you had six months ago left you feeling relaxed, nurtured and rejuvenated, but again—the money and the time would take away from what you give to your kids. And if/when you do go for the massage, you will be met with feelings of guilt. Where did this come from? Since when do we, as women, need to spend every minute and every dollar on our children?

Maybe this is not you, but it was me. And it rings true for many of my clients and other moms I've talked to. For me, it started the moment I became a mom. For some reason I felt I had to do it all—alone. I knew I married a great guy, but I did every nursing around the clock for what felt like an eternity. He offered that I could pump and he could bottle feed our daughter, but pumping felt like extra work and I felt like I was supposed to do it all. So, nine times out of ten, I declined his offer.

Was I being a control freak? Maybe. But maybe it was the mom guilt that drove me to make these decisions. These early months of parenting set the stage for me—I never quite knew how much I had to do by myself and what I could delegate. At times, I pushed away other people's offers to help. I felt limited by my own guilt.

Looking back, I take full ownership that it was my issue. It took having a health crash for me to learn to accept help. By that point I had no choice but to accept help because my body gave out and I was too depleted to do it all myself even if I tried! There were a few weeks that I could barely get out of bed because I was so exhausted and weak. During this time, my husband did all the childcare, my friends helped with grocery shopping, and I accepted help in the form of talk therapy.

It's okay to accept help *now,* before a health crash. You don't have to wait until your body breaks down like mine did. If a friend or family member offers to watch your kids—say yes!

People love to help. Allow them to give you that gift of feeling helpful. And if people aren't stepping forward to help, it's okay for you to ask. It's okay for you to ask your husband to help with errands, cooking, laundry, cleaning, and childcare, and it's okay for you to take a night off from parenting to go out with your girlfriends. It's okay for you to take time for exercise and the things that bring you joy. You need it and you deserve it.

> "When you put yourself first, your kids thrive."

-Kelly Danielle (Life Coach)

Gather more parenting tools. I'll be honest. I have often wished I had an instruction manual for this parenting gig. Prior to being a mom, I had a vision of what I hoped motherhood would be. That vision was idyllic. I will confess—I had almost zero experience with babies other than babysitting for a family with two young kids during my high school years. The family seemed perfect—a mom and dad, an older sister, and a younger brother. The two kids listened to my every word, they never fought, and it was the easiest and most fun job ever! So when it came time to start my own family, I thought it would be just the same.

The day my first child was born was magical. I was overjoyed--my dream of becoming a mom had come true. She was the most perfect, chubby little baby I had ever seen. The first week of motherhood was great. She ate, she slept, she pooped. It was exactly as I had read in the parenting books.

But then the colic started. And the nursing problems started. And my anxiety crept in. And then it was time to return to work, yet that was the last thing I wanted to do right then. I became torn between what I wanted to do and what I felt like I "should do." I didn't know what I should do anymore. Where was my rule book? Where was my parenting book for this colic that seemed never-ending?

We got through it, though. By her first birthday, my husband, daughter, and I felt like a happy little unit. Eventually we decided to expand our family, and with the birth of our beautiful son, I knew our family was complete.

Fast-forward a couple years, and parenting felt messy. It felt chaotic. It did not feel like it did when I babysat those two adorable angels. Why weren't my kids listening to me? What was I doing wrong?

I read more books. I observed my friends interacting with their kids. I noticed my teacher friends had a different skill set from mine. I learned from them, and I shared what I was learning with my husband (probably not always in the kindest way or at the most opportune times). But things still felt more stressful in the parenting department than I liked to admit.

My husband agreed to take a parenting class with me.

It was a DVD we could watch at home. We tried some of the techniques. Some worked for our "spirited" daughter, but other techniques didn't. And on some level, some of the techniques from this DVD felt a bit disrespectful, honestly.

Then one day I stumbled across another parenting program—it showed up in my Facebook newsfeed. *Positive Parenting Solutions*. Maybe it's been in your newsfeed, too? My husband and I watched a free webinar together. It was exactly what I was looking for—simple tactics that we could implement right away. We signed up for the program that day.

Watching the short videos and implementing the techniques took discipline--it took time out of our already busy and chaotic life. It required effort to change our actions, our words, and our reactions with our kids. But the tools made sense and they felt respectful. They gave my husband and me a common "rule book" to parent by. Little by little, we felt empowered, calm, and we were seeing results.

It has now been four years since starting this program, and we still use the tools and techniques daily. We continue to do weekly family meetings that have a simple agenda and leave each family member feeling uplifted. Check out this parenting program at www.positiveparentingsolutions.com.

Parenting requires ongoing learning and adjustment of (unrealistic) expectations. I am a huge believer that we were never meant to parent in isolation. I strongly suggest that you find ways to spend time with other moms and other families.

Mom intuition. Again, there's no rule book for parenting or for life. There is no shortage of advice coming from others—including your parents, friends, strangers, and even me. This advice is almost always well-meaning, but ultimately you know your kids and your life situation better than anyone. If you're unsure of what to do in a parenting situation, it can be helpful to gather information—facts, stories, advice, etc. But ultimately, trust you inner guidance in making decisions—big or small. Just like your body was designed to heal, you were given special instincts as a mother. This intuitive gift is like a muscle that, with practice, becomes stronger. What is your intuition guiding you to do (or not do)? Start listening…

A SPECIAL SECTION FOR WOMEN WITH ANXIETY

I am no stranger to anxiety. I lived with mild to moderate anxiety for twenty years and I now consider myself to be recovered. I experienced general anxiety in social situations, I often had trouble turning off my thoughts at bedtime, and I even had panic attacks when I had to speak in public. These days, though, I feel at ease in most social situations, I'm able relax my mind at bedtime, and I've learned to love public speaking.

How did I heal? It was a long process that took consistent effort, but my steps were simpler than you might expect. In addition to the "nourish to flourish toolkit" outlined in this book, I discovered these additional tools along the way:

Anxiety Relief Tools

1. **4-7-8 breathing:** I discussed this earlier in the book and it's worth mentioning again. Please look online for a video of Dr. Andrew Weil teaching this technique. This technique takes one minute and is most effective when practiced at least twice a day.

2. **Magnesium:** Magnesium is a mineral that people often call "the relaxation mineral." I first discovered this while recovering from my health crash, specifically a product called Natural Calm, made by Natural Vitality. It's magnesium citrate powder that you mix with warm water and drink. Many

people feel anxiety relief within minutes of taking it. It also helps improve sleep. There are *many* great supplements that can help relieve anxiety, help heal the gut, help reduce inflammation, and more. Supplements are outside the scope of this book; however, it is something that an experienced health coach and functional medicine practitioner can help you with.

3. **Barefoot yoga in my backyard:** During my health crash recovery, I discovered that yoga had an immediate calming effect for me. I had read about yoga and I knew a few poses that I'd learned here and there during my physical therapy career. As part of my personal prescription, I committed to doing five minutes of barefoot yoga every day. It helped me feel grounded, relaxed, and "less in my head" and more in my body. There are so many options for yoga—videos, classes, etc. Try a few and see what you like.

4. **Nature:** I noticed that when I got into nature, even just at the park by my house, I felt calmer. This feeling magnified when I went to the woods or to the beach, so I started to plan "nature adventures" with my family. Looking at giant redwood trees, watching birds soar, soaking my feet in a lake, standing barefoot in the sand. Each of these experiences delivered a sense of calm. The same is true for my clients. Some refer to this time in nature as "nature bathing," "forest bathing," or "nature resets." How do

you feel in nature? What effect does it have on your mind, body, and spirit? How can you build that into your day, week, or month?

5. **Lighten the load:** I began to look at all the things on my plate, i.e. my list of responsibilities, commitments, obligations, etc. It felt overwhelming in my head and when I wrote it down, it was still overwhelming. But little by little I have simplified it. I want you to do the same. Write it all down--I'm sure it's a long list. Really think about each item. Are there commitments that are no longer serving you? Are there things you can let go? Are there things you can ask for help with? I know this is hard, but if you want to feel better, I encourage you work on these things.

6. **Are you highly sensitive?** During health coaching school, I had some *aha* moments about the anxiety I had experienced for twenty years. I learned about the terms "highly sensitive person" and "empath." Highly sensitive people feel emotions more intensely than the average person—the happy emotions feel really happy and the sad feelings feel deeply sad. An empath is a person who is highly empathetic and easily can put themselves in another person's shoes, so to speak. An empath feels other people's physical and emotional pain. Are you highly sensitive? Are you an empath? I discovered that I'm both. So, my aha moment was that a lot of the anxiety I have felt in my lifetime

was not even my own; it belonged to others but, as a highly empathetic person, I felt it. On some level, I felt the pain that my physical therapy patients felt. I felt the pain of my family members—especially emotional pain. This is human, but if it is excessive, it can be harmful to one's health.

It took a lot of self-reflection and talk therapy, but I've since learned to set better boundaries. The idea of setting boundaries has been extremely helpful. I've learned how to help people without draining my own energy. I still sense other people's emotional pain, but now I'm aware that it's their pain and not my own. I also created an analogy to help me cope: if a family member, friend, or client is stuck at the bottom of a well, I will throw them a rope and give them instructions for how to climb out, but I won't let myself fall down in the well with them.

7. **You can only control you.** This was another *aha* moment for me that I learned in my healing journey: You can't choose everything in your life and you can't control others' words or actions, but you can choose how you react. Ultimately, you can only control yourself--your choices, your actions, your reactions.

8. **Do you worry about the future?** Anxiety is living in the future and believing that it's worse than right now. Your mind often plays out worst-case

scenarios. It robs you of the present moment. Additionally, these negative thoughts fill your body with a cascade of stress hormones—in essence, your body and mind experience the emotions of the negative event even though it hasn't happened. If you catch yourself worrying, try to flip your thoughts into positive ones. If you're safe in the present moment, remind yourself of that. It isn't always easy, but it can be done. I hope that after reading this book, you feel more empowered that you can change your life for the better. Your tomorrows can be better than your today.

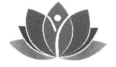

Part 3: Heal

This section will guide you to write and implement your personal prescription so that you can reclaim your health and happiness.

A healthy life begins with healthy habits.

Are you ready to implement what you have learned in this book? Reading this book is a great start, but changing your thoughts and your actions is where the magic happens. In this part of the book, I'll guide you through choosing your action steps.

In order to change your current reality, you must take full responsibility moving forward. You're responsible for your thoughts, your actions, and your reactions--not those of others—only you. Moving forward, you are in control of what interventions you choose, what food you eat, what you say "yes" to, and what you say "no" to. You are now becoming a "citizen scientist." You're trying different ways of eating, different ways of setting boundaries, different ways of thinking, different ways of nourishing yourself—and while you do this, you're gathering data. This data is unique to *you*. You'll begin to discover which foods work best for you, which things bring you joy, which bedtime routine works for you. You'll also learn what *doesn't* work for you. With this data, you can make educated choices to help you live your best life.

Does this sound scary or intimidating? Change can be scary for some people. And taking time for self-care is uncomfortable for many women. It may feel selfish for you. Please take baby steps. But keep putting one foot in front of the other, and you'll begin to see progress. Please know that self-care is an act of self-love. You were taught to love others—but were you taught to love yourself? I want you to love others and love yourself. Speak to yourself and care for yourself as you would your best friend or your child.

The more you nourish, the more you will flourish.

WRITE YOUR PERSONAL PRESCRIPTION

Please answer the following questions. This will guide Week 1. Use the form in Appendix B for Weeks 2-6. Set achievable action steps for each week. Celebrate all of your accomplishments in the next six weeks, whether big or small. Every step in the right direction counts.

Step 1: What *aha* lessons from Part 1 of the book resonated most with you? Refer to p. 52.

_____

_____

_____

_____

_____

Step 2: *Why* is good health important to you? What will better health allow you to do? How will achieving good health change your life? Knowing your "why" will help you persevere in your journey to better health. Good health *is not* a destination. Instead, good health is a vehicle; it allows you to live your life on your terms. In the space provided, please write your "why."

_____

_____

_____

_____

_____

Step 3: Visualize Success. What are your health and wellness goals? You must acknowledge where you are now and decide where you want to go in order to guide your choices moving forward. Create a vision for your life six months from now. How will you look and feel? Describe it. Get specific. Write it in the space below.

Visualize twice daily and attach joy and positive emotion to this visualization. Write a description of this visualization and place it on your mirror or put it on your nightstand. You must review it every morning upon waking up and every evening before going to sleep.

Date six months from today: _____
Describe the detailed visualization here:

_____

_____

_____

_____

_____

_____

_____

Step 4: Nourish with Food. Refer to page 77-78 and choose one action step that you will take to improve your nutrition in the next week.

_____

Step 5: Nourish with Water. Refer to page 82 and choose one action step that you can take in the next week.

_____

Step 6: Nourish with Sleep. Refer to p. 88 and choose one action step that you can implement in the next week.

_____

Step 7: Nourish with Movement. Refer to p. 96 and choose one action step that you can do in the next week. How and where can you incorporate movement into your week? Start with something small and achievable.

_____

Step 8: Nourish with Mindset. Review the mindset tips on p. 105-106. Begin a gratitude practice. Will you write/record three things per day, or simply think about them? Where in your day will you build this into your routine? For example, you might practice gratitude first thing upon waking up, or while brushing your teeth, or before bed.

_____

Step 9: Nourish with Joy. Review the tips on increasing joy on p. 113. What are three things that bring you joy? Start to think about how you can incorporate these things into your life.

3 things that bring me joy:

1. _____

2. _____

3. _____

Step 10: Accountability. In Part 1 of the book, we discussed a "healing team." You're taking full responsibility in your journey; however, you do not have to do this alone. Instead, I strongly encourage that you build a healing team; find a few people who support your quest for better health. The other key ingredient to your success is accountability. I suggest that you enlist a friend to join you on this journey. Each of you can read this book and fill out this worksheet to create your "personal prescription." Start by committing to six weeks. You then can schedule a time each week to check in with each other. A one-hour call works best. This way you can each have thirty minutes to focus on your own journeys. Gently and lovingly (and firmly) hold each other accountable for your chosen action steps. Then gradually move forward, supporting each other along the way.

My accountability partner is: _____

Time/Day that we will talk each week is: _____

_____

Put the six sessions on your calendar. Make it a priority. You are helping yourself and your friend.

At the end of the six weeks, celebrate your successes and create a plan moving forward. You may be able to spread out the calls to every other week or even once a month.

DO YOU WISH TO ACCELERATE YOUR CHANGE PROCESS?

If you want professional support on your journey, consider working with a health coach or functional medicine doctor. Make sure that you choose a provider who is a good fit for you. With the right provider, you'll feel validated, respected, supported, and empowered.

As a health coach, I recognize that each of my clients is at a different starting point and they each have different goals. I provide personalized care to help discover food and lifestyle choices that work best for each person. I guide my clients to make gradual, lifelong changes that allow them to reach their health and life goals. The results that my clients experience are profound and life changing. If you would like to learn more about my private health coaching services, please visit me at www.SimplyBalancedWellness.com.

"The greatest wealth is health."

-Virgil

CONCLUSION

I'm so glad you joined me with an open mind and an open heart as you read this handbook. The principles I shared with you are based in functional medicine. As I mentioned earlier, functional medicine addresses the underlying causes of disease, using a systematic and scientific approach, with the patient and the practitioner in a therapeutic partnership. This root cause approach to restoring health integrates traditional western medicine with nutrition and lifestyle changes; additionally, a functional medicine practitioner utilizes special lab tests to further tailor a program unique to the needs of each individual. "Appendix C" includes a list of my favorite functional medicine books that are specific to different medical conditions. Please take a look to discover books that can further help you and those you care about.

I wrote this handbook to inspire and support you in reclaiming your health and happiness. My fifteen-year career as a physical therapist gave me insight into the pros and cons of the traditional western medical system. This system thrives in some areas (like acute and trauma care), but is failing to help people reverse chronic health conditions. Using the functional medicine foundation of nutrition and lifestyle, I have successfully helped myself, my family, and my clients. This has been the most exciting few years of my life. I'm thrilled to share this information!

I encourage you to restore balance in areas of your life

that may have been out of balance. As a reminder, the key areas discussed in this book include nourishing with food, water, sleep, movement, mindset, and joy. The more you nourish these areas of your life, the more you will flourish. Healthy habits create a healthy life. The changes are often simple, but "simple" does not necessarily mean "easy." This process requires consistent effort and time. I know that you can do this. You are worth it. You deserve to feel better so you can live better. The best is yet to come!

With deepest gratitude and love,

Lauren Bahr

"Create the highest, grandest vision for your life, because you become what you believe."

-Oprah Winfrey

APPENDIX A
YOUR PERSONAL PRESCRIPTION:

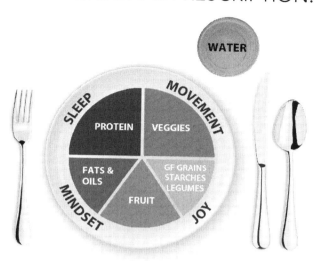

Ready, Set, Heal

Instructions: Please answer the following questions. This will guide Week 1. Use the form in Appendix B for Weeks 2-6. Set achievable action steps for each week. Celebrate all of your accomplishments in the next six weeks, whether big or small. Every step in the right direction counts.

Step 1: What *aha* lessons from Part 1 of the book resonated most with you? Refer to p. 52.

_____

_____

_____

_____

_____

Step 2: *Why* is good health important to you? What will better health allow you to do? How will achieving good health change your life? Knowing your "why" will help you persevere in your journey to better health. Good health *is not* a destination. Instead, good health is a vehicle; it allows you to live your life on your terms. In the space provided, please write your "why."

_____

_____

_____

_____

_____

Step 3: Visualize Success. What are your health and wellness goals? You must acknowledge where you are now and decide where you want to go in order to guide your choices moving forward. Create a vision for your life six months from now. How will you look and feel? Describe it. Get specific. Write it in the space below.

Visualize twice daily and attach joy and positive emotion to this visualization. Write a description of this visualization and place it on your mirror or put it on your nightstand. You must review it every morning upon waking up and every evening before going to sleep.

Date six months from today: _____
Describe the detailed visualization here:

_____

_____

_____

_____

_____

_____

_____

Step 4: Nourish with Food. Refer to page 77-78 and choose one action step that you will take to improve your nutrition in the next week.

_____

Step 5: Nourish with Water. Refer to page 82 and choose one action step that you can take in the next week.

_____

Step 6: Nourish with Sleep. Refer to p. 88 and choose one action step that you can implement in the next week.

_____

Step 7: Nourish with Movement. Refer to p. 96 and choose one action step that you can do in the next week. How and where can you incorporate movement into your week? Start with something small and achievable.

_____

Step 8: Nourish with Mindset. Review the mindset tips on p. 105-106. Begin a gratitude practice. Will you write/record three things per day, or simply think about them? Where in your day will you build this into your routine? For example, you might practice gratitude first thing upon waking up, or while brushing your teeth, or before bed.

_____

Step 9: Nourish with Joy. Review the tips on increasing joy on p. 113. What are three things that bring you joy? Start to think about how you can incorporate these things into your life.

3 things that bring me joy:

1. _____

2. _____

3. _____

Step 10: Accountability. In Part 1 of the book, we discussed a "healing team." You're taking full responsibility in your journey; however, you do not have to do this alone. Instead, I strongly encourage that you build a healing team; find a few people who support your quest for better health. The other key ingredient to your success is accountability. I suggest that you enlist a friend to join you on this journey. Each of you can read this book and fill out this worksheet to create your "personal prescription." Start by committing to six weeks. You then can schedule a time each week to check in with each other. A one-hour call works best. This way you can each have thirty minutes to focus on your own journeys. Gently and lovingly (and firmly) hold each other accountable for your chosen action steps. Then gradually move forward, supporting each other along the way.

My accountability partner is: _____

Time/Day that we will talk each week is: _____

_____

Put the six sessions on your calendar. Make it a priority. You are helping yourself and your friend.

At the end of the six weeks, celebrate your successes and create a plan moving forward. You may be able to spread out the calls to every other week or even once a month.

APPENDIX B
WEEKLY SELF-ASSESSMENT

Instructions: Use this form for weeks 2-6. Complete this form prior to meeting with your accountability partner. During your discussion, allow each person to have thirty minutes for sharing their accomplishments and their challenges. The listener's job is to provide encouragement, support, and accountability, while withholding judgement. Please provide a safe space for each other to feel heard and supported. Enjoy the journey!

NAME: _____ DATE: _____

In each of the following areas, make note of what went well in the past week:

Food: _____

Water: _____

Sleep: _____

Movement: _____

Mindset: _____

Joy: _____

My challenges in the past week:

_____

_____

_____

_____

_____

My focus areas for the next week are:

1. _____

2. _____

3. _____

APPENDIX C
RECOMMENDED RESOURCES

Connect with me:

- Visit my website: www.SimplyBalancedWellness.com to learn more about my health coaching services and/or sign up for my monthly newsletter for healthy living hacks and simple recipes.

- Visit my Facebook page at https://www.facebook.com/LaurenBahrWellness

- For speaking engagements, email me at Lauren@simply-balancedwellness.com

TED Talks:

- Terry Wahls, "Minding Your Mitochondria"

- Lissa Rankin, "Is There Scientific Proof We Can Heal Ourselves"

Functional Medicine Books:

- Grain Brain, by David Perlmutter, MD

- Mind over Medicine, by Lissa Rankin, MD

- Food: What the Heck Should I Eat? By Mark Hyman, MD

- Eat Fat, Get Thin, by Mark Hyman, MD

- Heal Your Pain Now, by Joe Tatta, DPT, CNS

- The Anti-Anxiety Food Solution, by Trudy Scott, CN

- The Adrenal Thyroid Revolution, by Aviva Romm, MD

- The Immune System Recovery Plan, by Susan Blum, MD, MPH

- The Hormone Cure, by Sara Gottfried, MD

- Dirty Genes, by Dr. Ben Lynch

- Mind Over Meds, by Andrew Weil, MD

- A Mind of Your Own: The Truth About Depression and How Women Can Heal Their Bodies to Reclaim Their Lives, by Kelly Brogan, MD

- How to Make Disease Disappear, by Dr. Rangan Chatterjee

- Healing the New Childhood Epidemics: Autism, ADHD, Asthma, and Allergies: The Groundbreaking Program for the 4-A Disorders, by Kenneth Bock and Cameron Stauth

Documentary:

- Heal Documentary: Change Your Mind. Change Your Body. Change Your Life, by Deepak Chopra, MD, Dr. Michael Beckwith, and Kelly Noonan Gores.

REFERENCES

Blum, S. (2013). *The Immune System Recovery Plan*. Simon & Shuster.

Hyman, M. (2018). *Food: What the heck should I eat?* New York: Little, Brown and Company.

Lynch, B. (2018). *Dirty genes: A breakthrough program to treat the root cause of illness and optimize your health*. New York, NY: HarperOne.

National Center for Health Statistics. (2017, August 15). Retrieved June 9, 2018, from https://www.cdc.gov/nchs/products/databriefs/db283.htm

Overweight & Obesity Statistics. (2017, August 01). Retrieved June 9, 2018, from https://www.niddk.nih.gov/health-information/health-statistics/overweight-obesity

Romm, A. J. (2017). *The adrenal thyroid revolution*. New York, NY: HarperOne.

Video: Dr. Weil's Breathing Exercises: 4-7-8 Breath. (2017, September 20). Retrieved July 9, 2018, from https://www.drweil.com/videos-features/videos/breathing-exercises-4-7-8-breath/)

What does organic mean? (n.d.). Retrieved July 7, 2018, from

https://www.ewg.org/research/organic-within-reach/
what-does-organic-mean#.W1sul9JKjlU

33403530R00084

Made in the USA
Middletown, DE
14 January 2019